T0284319

Besides being beautiful little hand-sized objects themselves, showcasing exceptional writing, the wonder of these books is that they exist at all ... Uniformly excellent, engaging, thought-provoking, and informative."

Jennifer Bort Yacovissi, *Washington Independent Review of Books*

... edifying and entertaining ... perfect for slipping in a pocket and pulling out when life is on hold."

Sarah Murdoch, *Toronto Star*

For my money, Object Lessons is the most consistently interesting nonfiction book series in America."

PopMatters

Though short, at roughly 25,000 words apiece, these books are anything but slight."

Marina Benjamin, *New Statesman*

[W]itty, thought-provoking, and poetic ... These little books are a page-flipper's dream."

John Timpane, *The Philadelphia Inquirer*

OBJECTLESSONS

A book series about the hidden lives of ordinary things.

Series Editors:

Ian Bogost and Christopher Schaberg

In association with

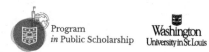

Program
in Public Scholarship

Washington
University in St.Louis

BOOKS IN THE SERIES

Air Conditioning by Hsuan L. Hsu
Alarm by Alice Bennett
Barcode by Jordan Frith
Bicycle by Jonathan Maskit
Bird by Erik Anderson
Blackface by Ayanna Thompson
Blanket by Kara Thompson
Blue Jeans by Carolyn Purnell
Bookshelf by Lydia Pyne
Bread by Scott Cutler Shershow
Bulletproof Vest by Kenneth R. Rosen
Burger by Carol J. Adams
Cell Tower by Steven E. Jones
Cigarette Lighter by Jack Pendarvis
Coffee by Dinah Lenney
Compact Disc by Robert Barry
Doctor by Andrew Bomback
Dust by Michael Marder
Doll Maria Teresa Hart
Driver's License by Meredith Castile
Drone by Adam Rothstein
Earth by Jeffrey Jerome Cohen and Linda T. Elkins-Tanton
Egg by Nicole Walker
Email by Randy Malamud
Environment by Rolf Halden
Exit by Laura Waddell
Eye Chart by William Germano
Fat by Hanne Blank
Fake by Kati Stevens
Football by Mark Yakich
Gin by Shonna Milliken Humphrey
Glitter by Nicole Seymour
Glass by John Garrison
Golf Ball by Harry Brown
Grave Allison C. Meier
Hair by Scott Lowe
Hashtag by Elizabeth Losh
High Heel by Summer Brennan
Hood by Alison Kinney
Hotel by Joanna Walsh
Hyphen by Pardis Mahdavi
Jet Lag by Christopher J. Lee
Luggage by Susan Harlan
Magazine by Jeff Jarvis
Magnet by Eva Barbarossa
Mask by Sharrona Pearl

Mushroom by Sara Rich
Newspaper by Maggie Messitt
Ocean by Steve Mentz
Office by Sheila Liming
OK by Michelle McSweeney
Password by Martin Paul Eve
Perfume by Megan Volpert
Personal Stereo by Rebecca Tuhus-Dubrow
Phone Booth by Ariana Kelly
Pill by Robert Bennett
Political Sign by Tobias Carroll
Potato by Rebecca Earle
Pregnancy Test by Karen Weingarten
Questionnaire by Evan Kindley
Recipe by Lynn Z. Bloom
Refrigerator by Jonathan Rees
Remote Control by Caetlin Benson-Allott
Rust by Jean-Michel Rabaté
Scream by Michael J. Seidlinger
Sewer by Jessica Leigh Hester
Shipping Container by Craig Martin
Shopping Mall by Matthew Newton
Signature by Hunter Dukes
Silence by John Biguenet
Skateboard by Jonathan Russell Clark
Snake by Erica Wright
Sock by Kim Adrian
Souvenir by Rolf Potts
Spacecraft by Timothy Morton
Space Rover by Stewart Lawrence Sinclair
Sticker by Henry Hoke
Stroller by Amanda Parrish Morgan
Traffic by Paul Josephson
Tree by Matthew Battles
Trench Coat by Jane Tynan
Tumor by Anna Leahy
TV by Susan Bordo
Veil by Rafia Zakaria
Waste by Brian Thill
Whale Song by Margret Grebowicz
Wine Meg Bernhard
(Forthcoming)
Concrete Stephen Parnell
Fist by nelle mills
Fog by Stephen Sparks
Train by A. N. Devers

Mask

SHARRONA PEARL

BLOOMSBURY ACADEMIC
NEW YORK • LONDON • OXFORD • NEW DELHI • SYDNEY

BLOOMSBURY ACADEMIC
Bloomsbury Publishing Inc
1385 Broadway, New York, NY 10018, USA
50 Bedford Square, London, WC1B 3DP, UK
29 Earlsfort Terrace, Dublin 2, Ireland

BLOOMSBURY, BLOOMSBURY ACADEMIC and the Diana logo are trademarks
of Bloomsbury Publishing Plc

First published in the United States of America 2024

Cover design: Alice Marwick

Library of Congress Cataloging-in-Publication Data
Names: Pearl, Sharrona, author.
Title: Mask / Sharrona Pearl.
Description: New York : Bloomsbury Academic, 2024. | Series: Object lessons | Includes
bibliographical references and index. | Summary: "Mask will explore the long history of masking,
asking who and what we seek to protect through different forms of masks"–Provided by publisher.
Identifiers: LCCN 2023042530 (print) | LCCN 2023042531 (ebook) | ISBN 9798765102404 (paper-
back) | ISBN 9798765102411 (ebook) | ISBN 9798765102428 (pdf)
Subjects: LCSH: Masks–Social aspects. | Masks–Symbolic aspects.
Classification: LCC GN419.5 .P43 2024 (print) | LCC GN419.5 (ebook) | DDC 391.4/3409–dc23/
eng/20240129
LC record available at https://lccn.loc.gov/2023042530
LC ebook record available at https://lccn.loc.gov/2023042531

ISBN: PB: 979-8-7651-0240-4
       ePDF: 979-8-7651-0242-8
       eBook: 979-8-7651-0241-1

Series: Object Lessons

Typeset by Deanta Global Publishing Services, Chennai, India
Printed and bound in Great Britain.

To find out more about our authors and books visit www.bloomsbury.com
and sign up for our newsletters.

CONTENTS

Introduction 1

1 My Mask Rules, Often Broken 11

2 Physiognomy 17

3 Feature/Bug: Multivalence 23

4 History: Not of Socks 27

5 Performing as Protection 35

6 Freedom and Constraint: Whose
Trust Matters 39

7 Medical Masks and the Covid Elephant 51

8 Violence and the Masks of War 59

9 No Way to Hide 63

10 Villain/Hero: V'nahafoch hu 69

11 Superheroes, or Who Watches the Watchers 81

12 The Eyes Have It: Face Facemasks and Looking Like Ourselves 87

13 Exposure 97

Acknowledgments 105
Bibliography 107
Index 109

INTRODUCTION

When I was four years old, I was pulled out of my junior kindergarten class in Toronto, terrifyingly, to report to the office. It turns out I was selected to participate in a brief television interview for a show called *Just Kidding* along with two other kids, Bradley C. and Ilana Z. They were there because they were extremely charming and precocious; I was there because my mother was friends with the school principal. The conceit of the show, pioneered in 1968 by Art Linkletter and since revisited many times in multiple formats, was to capture the sweet and silly things that young children say, often naively. Shameless pandering with a dash of cynicism, wrapped up in an adorable and ideally hilarious package. (I think the show lasted two seasons.) In my 30 seconds of fame, for which I later thrillingly received a check for $50 (CDN), I patiently explained, as per my prompt, the difference between a robber and a thief. The robber, I knowledgably shared, "wears a mask around his eyes."

A four-year-old would be unlikely to know that robbery includes stealing with the use of force, while theft is absent any acts of violence or aggression. (A lot of non-four-year-olds are also unlikely to know this distinction. Did you?) It's not surprising that I reached for an easy visual signifier: the cartoonish black mask that I probably saw on costumes and in advertisements, along with a sinister slinking gait and a full black sack slung over the perpetrator's shoulder. (As a kid who grew up keeping kosher, my closest relationship to the Hamburglar—the obvious referent here—was in TV commercials as something distant and unrelated to my life.) To me, at four, being blindsided by an impossible ask, I turned to the most obvious point of distinction I could imagine: one category had an exposed face, and the other did not. The mask was a powerful visual way to assign difference where no meaningful difference existed for me. The mask marked one type of person from another. The mask of the "robber" made it a different kind of thing to the bare-eyed "thief." And of course to me, the one covering their face was worse. The one covering their face was the real one to fear.

Given that robbers are the ones who use force, I was perhaps not far off in my gut reaction. And I was not wrong that masks can sometimes tell us quite a lot: about the person wearing them, about their cultural context, about what they wish to hide and what they wish to reveal, about what others wish them to hide. Masks can also sometimes tell us about what people reveal while attempting to hide, and about how others feel about those wearing the masks. Robbers, to my 4-year-old self, wore masks to protect themselves from detection and persecution in the course of committing a crime. Hiding is one way that masks offers protection. It's not the only one.[1]

---

[1]Another anecdote: when I was discussing this project with my wonderful editors at Bloomsbury Academic Press, my husband had the great suggestion of asking them to send me a sample of other books in the *Object Lessons* series. I'd already sent in my proposal, and I think I already had the contract, so I wasn't imagining these books to change too much in what I would write, but instead give me a sense of the style, flavor, and range of the other objects and the lessons they brought to bear. On my shelf are now books about socks and remote controls and hoods and hotels. And they differ a great deal: the one about socks, for example, is really about socks. It tells you the history of socks, when they were first discovered (around 5500 years ago, in case you are interested, and if you are really interested you should read the book!), different techniques in creating socks, who wears socks and why. The book on hoods is about various kinds of hoods, but also about structural racism, concealment, and the stakes for wearing hoodies in the contemporary United States. (Read that one too.) I started to get a sense that these books about objects were really about those objects: their history, their cultural context, their use, and their meaning. This all made sense.

Then I read the book about hotels. And let me be clear: I was extremely interested to learn about hotels. I *love* hotels. I love curling up in a big, pre-made bed and doing something illicit like eating takeout food while lying in a sea of too many overstuffed pillows. I love their sterile furnishings and the sense that I could be anywhere and nowhere at all. I love being all by myself for a bit. I used to watch a steamy British television show called *Hotel Babylon* about the seedy underside of hotels, until I couldn't find it streaming in the US anymore. So I really quite wanted to read about hotels. And look, the book is sort of about hotels. But it's also a Freudian excavation of the meaning of home, a deep dive into dreams, and a literary conjuring of the ache where belonging once was.

And then I realized: this book could be about *absolutely anything*. Obviously it has to be about masks—I want it to be about masks—but where I go with it is entirely up to me. So buckle up, friends; we are about to take

Protection is (at least) a two-way street. Masks can protect the wearer, and masks can protect others from the one wearing the mask. We know this now, in a grounded and global way, in the context of airborne respiratory illnesses like, say, Covid-19. Others have known this in a very different way. Consider the muhapatti, the white mouth covering worn by some sects within the Jain religion. These masks serve a number of functions, including protecting sacred texts, images, and ritual objects from saliva. They are also a manifestation of and key aide toward the realization of the central Jain principle of ahimsa—the repudiation of violence in all aspects of existence. The muhapatti providers a barrier that limits the wearer from inhaling small airborne organisms and causing their death, protecting both the organisms from the violence and the wearer from committing it and betraying a sacred philosophy. Both practical and symbolic in its protection, the muhapatti limits the violation of ahimsa for the wearer while reminding them of its centrality. And of course, this kind of mask, publicly visible and religiously meaningful, tells those who see it something about the wearer's beliefs, culture, and way of being in the world. It protects multiple entities; it conceals

---

a deep dive into not just the object of the mask and its meaning in culture and context, but what, really, concealment and revelation mean to me. And I didn't know this going in, but it makes a whole lot of sense that concealment and revelation are, to me, all about religion, and ritual, and the search for transcendence and meaning. And also, television.

that which it covers; it reveals information which might otherwise be unknown.

There are parades of masks across cultures and religious traditions. And there are parades of masks that are marked in historical memory for what they obscure, and what they lay bare. January 6, 2020: in Washington DC, a day of insurrection, of (even more) loss of innocence. A day of destruction and desecration. And also, a day of masks: medical masks for the government workers following mandated protocols; masks of anonymity and aggression for the armed insurrectionists yelling "don't tread on me" on their faces even as they hide who they are; gas masks and respirators and face shields designed to minimize that chaos, the casualties, and the cost. The many masks were a collection of historical contingencies, offering protection against disease, chemical warfare, identification technologies, medical interventions and limitations. We can look to the particular constellation of masks of that moment to understand where we were in time in multiple ways: culturally, socially, and politically, even as all these different masks have long endured.

A robber's mask, like many technologies of identity obstruction, covers the space between the eyes. The Janian mask, like the Covid mask, like many technologies of transmission reduction, covers the mouth. The gas mask and the anonymity mask cover the entire face, precisely in order to obscure it. All these masks protect, as masks do. All conceal, as masks do. And, as that which conceals always does, if we know how to look and how to see what is and is not visible alongside one another, what is and is not explicit, what is and is not displayed—meaningfully and in ways symbolic and grounded, theoretical and practical, reveal.

Of course masks are all about concealment and revelation, which, in my rendering, means we'll talk about surveillance, submission, and protection. Which means we'll necessarily talk about the cultures of masks users. The through line here is that masking is about protection. *By looking at masking, we can see who and what we value as worth of protection.* That's pithy. And true. But the book is not just about that. The recent weaponization of the medical mask has infused it with multiple additional meanings on top of the many meanings that were already there: in addition to being a barrier for viral transmission, masks—and the wearing of them—became a very public marker of a range of political and epidemiological commitments. In this way, the medical mask itself and its use have become a proxy for politics. But masks also sometimes quite literally say things on their surfaces, conveying additional messages about the wearer beyond the fact that they are being worn.

This book is the story of the mask: as a historical entity, with multiple meanings and uses; as an idea, a way to think about what it means to conceal and reveal; as a tool, weaponized and strategically deployed; as an encapsulation of trust; as an extension of the self. Masks are everywhere, even if we didn't always notice them.[2] There are a lot of different kinds of masks, and a lot of different kinds of mask

---

[2] We notice masks now. Quick: try not to think of an elephant. Masks are now the elephant in the room that we can't not notice. I write this book and think about masks in the long shadow of the pandemic, which has narrowed the mask into a thing, ideally disposable, that fits over the nose and mouth and is worn mostly indoors and mostly by people who believe in the persistence and danger, and don't want to perpetuate the spread, of Covid-19. That group does not include everyone. (It never does.) This book is not about Covid. (This book is about Covid. It's actually impossible now to talk about masks outside that context. Even if I wished to write the mask version of the sock book, hewing closely to the mechanics and material culture and history of the mask as a rigidly defined object, it would still be about Covid. Given the enormous and truly life-changing and world-changing effects and implications of this most recent global pandemic, every mask is interpolated through the medical face covering as object, and all the meanings it enrolls. While I will discuss a variety of masks and mask meanings, they will all inevitably be filtered through what is for us maskiest of masks, the ur-meaning of masks, the mask through which all other masks are understood. I cannot say that every examination of masks will now always and forever be an examination of Covid masks, but I am fairly confident that this will be true at least for a little while. At least as long as there is Covid, which is going to be a long, long time.)

I could write an entire book about Covid masking. People already have! And more will! It could be entirely about the more specific interrelated stories of Covid masking, racism, and public health protection. It could get even more granular and think about the weaponization of masking and health during the pandemic, and it would still probably be too long. But this is going to be a more general reflection on masks as both object and symbol, while still being invested quite specifically in the material thing itself, or itselves. There are a lot of different kinds of masks, and the term and category are so capricious and multivalent that it runs the risk of meaning nothing at all.

stories. I could tell it in pictures. In materials. In rituals. In performances. In feelings and emotions and experiences. I could tell it in successes: the ones who got away, the ones who survived, the ones whose rituals brought transcendence, the ones who brought the house down. Or I could tell it in failures: the ones who got caught, the ones who died, the ones who remained mired in the prosaic, the ones whose performances were duds. And I could also say: even when the mask succeeded, there were also failures.

We will look at masks across a variety of interconnected domains, thinking about their roles in ritual and religion, performance and theatre, medicine, surveillance, and superhero stories. We'll look at the history of the mask as an object, a symbol, and a way of being in the world across different cultures and timeframes, exploring the overlap between ritual, performance, representation, and exposure. Across all spaces, we will consider the role of the mask as both concealing and revealing, asking how it then necessarily transforms both the wearers and those around them, bringing new entities into being. We will see that questions of trust and identity underlie so much of what's at stake in covering and uncovering our faces. The mask is often an extension of, and space for, identity, leading us to consider what the mask says about those who wear it and those who do not. We will think about the material culture of the mask: What is it made of? What can we know about its moment by how it is constructed? Is it accessible? What does it leave behind? We will look at manifestations of masks in film and television, exploring the way that narratives of trust, surveillance, concealment and revelation underlie these stories. We'll think about racism and religious oppression in masking narratives, thinking closely about who we trust behind their masks, and who we do not. As we discuss the role of the mask as a means of protection, concealment, and communication, we'll ask: who does it protect? Whom does it exclude?

There were always people left behind.

1 MY MASK RULES, OFTEN BROKEN

"All is discovered! Flee at once!"

—SIR ARTHUR CONAN DOYLE, PROBABLY

We don't know if Sir Arthur Conan Doyle really sent this message on a telegram to twelve prominent and respected community leaders, and we certainly don't know if—as the legend goes—they opened the notes, panicked, and immediately disappeared from public life. Printed in the *Strand* magazine in 1897, the likely apocryphal tale touches on some of our deepest fears about ourselves, and about those around us. We all have secrets. We all have something to hide. What may be significant and seemingly ruinous to one person could be minor to another, but that probably wouldn't stop the first person from doing what they could to prevent discovery. We all, in some way or another, conceal. We all, at times, wear masks. But what if the mask itself reveals? Or to put a finer point on it: what *does* the mask itself reveal?

To mask is to cover. To conceal. If we are all concealing, can we all be unmasked? Ask yourself: what do I have to hide? What am I hiding, and from whom? Or from what? Those are questions both big and trivial: we all must conceal a little. Or a lot. We all must protect ourselves. Constant exposure is raw and vulnerable and sensitive and unsustainable. This is a metaphor.

This is not a metaphor. We need to keep certain physicalbodilyvisceralstabitanditbleeds parts under wraps. Is clothing a mask? Roland Barthes said that mustaches are masks. Is that a metaphor? A beard can certainly hide what is known as a weak chin. (What kind of strength is in a chin? Can strong chins open jars? The vestiges of physiognomy appear in surprising places.) The thing is, if everything that covers is a mask, we can't really talk about masks as things anymore. It also stops being interesting. You don't want to read a book about tablecloths except maybe you do, and there might well be a tablecloths book in this series, and I bet there is plenty to say about tablecloths and embroidery and tapestry, so I take it back, but maybe it's better to say that you don't want to read a mask book about tablecloths, and I get that. I don't really want to write a mask book about tablecloths. I want to write a mask book about masks. First I have to figure out what a mask is, and for the purposes of this book at least, what it isn't. But this is an invention, because I'm going to leave out all kinds of mask-like things that do what masks do: cover; protect; conceal. Tablecloths do that. But I am less interested here in which tables we protect than which people we protect.

We also mask ourselves. Metaphorically, but also quite literally, with all kinds of physical masks that do all kinds of different things, from guarding against disease to providing barriers from injury to obscuring faces from detection to mimicking the faces of others. What they share in common with one another and with the metaphorical mask is protection. Masks serve to protect. From and for what, however, changes. We can look at masks to determine what needs protecting in a given time and place, who needs protecting, who deserves protecting, to whom protection is offered and afforded, and to whom it is not. So yes: the mask is of course a metaphor for hiding, repressing, misleading, obscuring, concealing, covering, maybe even colluding and collaborating. We mask feelings, and bruises, and pain, and experiences. We mask memories. We mask smells. We mask meaning. And we also mask our faces.

So, rule #1: We will talk about masks used by people. No tablecloths then, and no lawnmower covers and no paint.

Rule #2: We'll discuss only masks that are designed for and go on the face. I'm mostly a scholar of faces, and that's what I know about and want to write about. It's my book. In this case, I do (at least partly) make the rules.

Rule #3: The masks we discuss have to cover and conceal and protect. That's how I'm defining masks, at least for the community we—readers and writer—are creating around this book. So no bandages or clothing or hats. But remember that both masks and their concealment may be metaphors, so that still gives us a lot of leeway about ways to cover the face.

(Is a mask a prosthesis?)

Rule #4: Some fights will not be debated here. I will not be both-siding the Covid mask issue. Again, my book, my rules. I'll nuance it, some, by thinking about what is gained and what is lost by medical masking. The portrait artist, disability activist, and author Riva Lehrer writes movingly about her concept of "face hunger." She has longed throughout the pandemic, as a person and a portraitist, to see the bare and exposed and entire human face, both in moments of deep publicity and moments of the most bounded intimacy. She still always wore her mask. That doesn't mean that it hasn't been hard. There were (are) losses in masking, medical and otherwise. Some of those losses—of being able to identify someone, for example, or of easily spreading disease, or of leaving a vulnerable body part exposed—are deliberate, are the explicit goals of a given mask and its purpose, are a feature not a bug. Lehrer writes about performing her own face, consciously drawing attention up to control where others focus, and to perhaps stop them from focusing on her body by making them look at her face. There is, for many, a loss of identity, of a way of being with others, of a deep sense of self, with the loss of an exposed face. For others, there is relief in *not* performing the self, in not being told to smile more, in not having, for example, facial disfigurement always on display. It's a different kind of identity loss, and sometimes a welcome one. With a concealed face, other parts of the self can be exposed.

Other losses are an unfortunate side effect of a necessary intervention. Obscuring identity *is the point* with riot masks or face stockings worn by those committing crimes. The masked anonymity of your colleagues in the hallways at work or your health care practitioner is a difficult consequence of masks. One kind of mask is not the same as the other. A successful mask in one kind of context is a failure in another. Context matters. So does the kind of mask in question.

Rule #5: There are sanctioned masks like medical masks and sports masks and cold-weather masks and theatre masks and some religious masks (religion is complicated: we'll get to it, but for now, some religions are sanctioned and some are not in some places and not others). There are unsanctioned masks like face stockings. And there are masks that have been sanctioned at some points in time and not in others. Ku Klux Klan (*yimach shemam*, as we say in Hebrew: may their names be erased and may they be eradicated) masks were tacitly sanctioned when the crimes their wearers were committing were themselves tacitly sanctioned, and when those responsible for sanctions were often the same people as those committing the atrocities. If you don't really care to find out the identity of the murderer behind the mask, you aren't really all that fussed about the mask itself. The protection it offers is also for those looking for an excuse not to care. This may also be true now in terms of whose masking is criminalized, and whose unmasking is criminalized. That may be wrong. Masks are multivalent.

Masks are multivalent. Maybe there are no real rules. Maybe there is only history and experience and memory, which is, of course, a whole hell of a lot.

2 PHYSIOGNOMY

What can we see when we look at masks? What can we know? I'm a historian, and I'm trained to make arguments and claims. But life—and objects—are messy. I could tell a story about why mask wearing makes us uncomfortable, nervous, confused, restricted. We like to see people's faces because we think we know something about them based on how they look. We like to show people our faces because we like to communicate that we have nothing to hide. Or we like to control what it is we are hiding. And we think that is visible in the face. This dates back to the ancient practice of physiognomy, and the idea that the face is a way to access the human interior has manifested in divination, religion, portraiture, philosophy, ethics, and, in more modern manifestations, biological anthropology, racial profiling, and makeover television. The role of masks in obstructing access to the face, its features, and its expressions, is sometimes a feature and sometimes a bug. But it matters because the face matters. To write about the mask is, inevitably, to write about the face.

We say a great deal about ourselves with how we appear to others. The mask barrier can make us uncomfortable not just physically but because we cannot see the faces of others. And then, maybe, we cannot know them. Or we cannot know them as well as we might have. But masks say other things, or things other than our faces do. A medical mask has recently indicated a commitment to public health; a belief in science; a concern for others alongside oneself. (Not wearing a mask during the heart of the Covid-19 pandemic has also held some specific meanings.) But medical masks are only a small part of the story. Masks have a long history of doing all kinds of identity work.

The links between the face and identity—real and imagined (and of course the imagined is very, very real)—are strong and enduring. We look at people and imagine we know something about them. That's not a gut instinct, or not just: we are responding to all kind of deliberate and subconscious and accidental and historical and cultural and social cues that people manifest in their person. What we wear—what we choose to wear, what we can afford to wear, what we are mandated by our jobs or gender norms or religious affiliations or bodily comfort or political commitment to wear—can say something about who we are. How we speak says something. It's not always clear what. Accents can change; language conventions can vary; cadences are subject to a variety of historical, cultural, and biological factors. Our hairstyles, our skin (tone, clarity, smoothness), contain stories, multivalent and sometimes manipulated. Our faces do identity work, but are far from transparent.

That doesn't stop us from making judgments about people based on how they look, and based on what we see when we look at them, and based on what we imagine we see when we look at them. The age-old practice of physiognomy provides a deeply flawed, highly manipulable, very changeable, and totally aspirational set of guidelines about the meaning of the face. It's no surprise that physiognomy has endured in various forms, guises, and cultures from antiquity through today. From divination to portraiture, preaching to parable, etiquette manuals to business guidelines, social registers to communal characteristics, physiognomy has proven flexible and enduring. It's a neat little trick to judge someone based on how they look and infuse that judgment with a narrative of justification: it's not me, it's physiognomy!

While the practice dates back to pseudo-Aristotelean writings in antiquity, it has been used as a form of divination, a way for artists to represent character traits, and, from the late eighteenth century in the hands of Swiss Pastor Johann Caspar Lavater, a practice to sustain social hierarchies by infusing certain features with elite characteristics. For Lavater, physiognomy was a way to access the Divine. In keeping with Enlightenment principles that suggested studying nature as a way to understand and glorify the workings of the Creator, Lavater framed physiognomy as a way to access the obscured interior of humanity through the visible exterior. Throughout the nineteenth century, various practitioners tried to codify physiognomy into more rigorous systems that could be used to make sense of the people around them with numerous accessible physiognomical guidebooks and principles. In a famous example, Charles Darwin was almost denied passage on the *Beagle* for the trip that helped him define his theory of evolution; the captain of the ship, Robert Fitzroy, felt that Darwin's nose indicated a lack of the fortitude necessary to see such a rigorous journey through. (Honestly, if you read Darwin's journals from the trip, Fitzroy was sort of right.) While physiognomy could be used to imagine something about individuals à la Darwin's nose, it also became a descriptive mechanism for large groups, providing rhetoric around, say, what Jews looked like, or poor people looked like, or Irish people looked like, and what that said about them as a group. It didn't then and it doesn't now matter if such descriptions were right (they weren't and they aren't); the point is that it was easy and useful to think we can quickly assess who people are based only on the faces they show to the world, particularly in the nineteenth-century context of urbanization and industrialization. With so many more people to encounter so quickly in the teeming city streets, physiognomy was a useful shorthand in an increasingly global and inhabited world.

Even as we resist something so obviously contingent and biased and problematic, it's extremely seductive to imagine that we can access something so complicated and meaningful and invisible as the interior identity of others simply by looking at them. Is that why we don't trust people in masks? It's extremely annoying not to be able to see other people's faces. It creates a barrier: to intimacy, to relationships, to communication. When are we more private with others—in our homes, unmasked, divided by a screen on a video call? Or in the same place, bodily together, but divided by a mask? The notion of public and private has been in flux, which is one possible explanation for why, in the early days of pandemic Zoom meetings, so many people made so many mistakes and exposed so very much in the privacy of their own homes on very public screens. Those many and much-memed moments of exposure were mortifying for all involved, but they were absolutely authentic and unintended. These were moments in which nothing, absolutely nothing, tragically nothing, was hidden.

Isn't hiding, obscuring, covering, *bad*? There may be reasons for it—the pandemic is one good but not the only example—but as a general principle, don't we want things to be exposed? Some people do. Many, many people don't, but I guess that's kind of the point: the ones who wish their deeds to remain unknown are probably up to no good, or at least no good according to those in power, who may themselves be bad. I could list all kinds of exposed (and, errr, exposing) people who have violated rules, laws, and social contracts. I don't need to. You know who they are. And yeah: they are bad people. It's all kinds of good their misdeeds were unmasked. But we're not talking about them. Their masks did not cover their faces. And while their masks protected (them) and concealed (them) and covered (them), they are again metaphorical and again non-facial. That doesn't mean that all facial masks are good. Masks are multivalent: in meaning, and in kind. Some are good and some are bad and if you replace the word obscuring with protecting, it becomes a whole different discussion.

There are many kinds of masks, and they do many kinds of things. There are many kinds of faces, and the stakes for them being masks are quite different. We chafe (literally, sometimes) at mask-wearing because we like to see faces. We like to see expressions. We imagine we know something about people based on how they look, and we feel like we can more easily build relationships, remember those around us, experience intimacy, and forge connections when we are face-to-bared-face with others. We even make rules about not-masking as a way to insist on this face-to-face encounter, in order to more easily facilitate ways of knowing others, in order to more effectively surveil those around us. Or, some of those around us. There are people who are allowed to mask, whose trustworthiness is already assumed, whose covered faces are not sources of anxiety or concern. This isn't hyperbole. The anti-mask laws date back to the nineteenth century in the US (that's kind of long for this relatively young country) and did (and do) render masking illegal in many states in the union.

To write about the mask is, inevitably, to write about trust. What forms of trust does the mask engender and interrupt? What do we see when we look at masks? And what do we think we are missing?

Let's find out.

3 FEATURE/BUG

MULTIVALENCE

While masks are designed to protect something or someone, they often also obscure features, identity, expression, emotion. Sometimes that's the central feature of a mask. And sometimes, it's a bug. It all depends on the mask. And the wearer. And the context.

Consider the helmet/face mask worn by hockey goalies. (I add in the goalie's face mask to get around my rules, which the helmet alone would not satisfy. And also to include hockey: I'm Canadian, eh? While the mounting evidence about the prevalence of CTE and other traumatic brain injuries in professional athletes have made it impossible for me to enjoy watching most broadcast sports, you can't really ever take the Toronto out of the girl. Go Leafs! This is a largely futile statement so I feel comfortable making it.) While such a mask obscures identity (even as the sports jersey convention of last names reveals it) that's not it's point. It's a bug, not a feature. Unless, of course, the face mask is not being used for a hockey game. (I'm reminded here of the Jewish principle of *muksa*, which is, essentially, the designation assigned to any object or entity that cannot be touched on the Jewish sabbath because its use would violate traditional observance of the day. For example, it is forbidden to light a fire on the sabbath; matches or a lighter would be considered muksa and thus cannot be handled in case this leads to their use, accidental or otherwise. There is, however, an exception, a kind of work around: if the object's use is reassigned to something that would not violate observance prior to the sabbath, it can be so used for that purpose. The classic example is of a hammer, whose traditional use as a building implement is prohibited. It can be designated a doorstop prior to the sabbath and thus handled as part of this very specific and admittedly unlikely application. If that's too obscure, think instead of eggplants who meaning has shifted entirely in specific contexts. Or the pear: drawn by nineteenth-century French caricaturist Honoré Daumier to circumvent the rules against mocking images of monarch Louis Philippe, it became the king. Meanings can shift and take root and actually change the objects with which they are associated. And feature and bug are not always distinct.) Hockey goalie masks are to protect the wearer from pucks to the head, not to turn him into cult-horror villain Jason. (Cue stabbing gif.) But once the Jason factor emerges, it becomes part of the mask's meaning and purpose. The hammer becomes a doorstop.

Objects have multiple uses, some primary to their function and some ancillary, but the primary and the ancillary are shifting fields. A face mask may be primarily to protect the wearer from small, dangerously fast flying disks to the head, but can also serve as an excellent way to avoid identification. In both cases, the mask is shielding the face, but to entirely different ends. A balaclava (winter hat that includes a face covering) is an excellent way to protect the face from the elements, particularly while skiing or hiking in extreme weather. It's also yet another great way to keep people from seeing and identifying one's face. A hockey goalie may actually wish for their face to be visible, but the protective imperative supersedes the publicity one. There may be losses in peripheral vision that affect play. The inability to signal one's teammates by expression might have costs. On the other hand, perhaps there are athletic or even professional advantages to keeping one's face obscured. But none of these are the specific goal of this particular face mask.

Other masks work differently. The mask in its basic form is a face cover, but the meaning and actual details of its conferred protection varies wildly. Sometimes the masked are the heroes: athletes, performers, savers of lives. Sometimes they are the villains: law breakers, those seeking to cause harm to others. Sometimes, it's not clear: vigilantes, protestors, the hunted and the hunters. Once upon a time, the Ku Klux Klan wore masks to protect their identities, but that served largely to protect law enforcement from even pretending to try to prosecute them. The line between villain and hero changes. The line between protector and persecutor changes.

There are different kinds of protection. There are different kinds of people who need to be protected. There always have been. History may not repeat itself exactly, but it certainly can seem familiar.

4 HISTORY

NOT OF SOCKS

Once upon a time, likely around 9000 BCE, there was a stone mask. It went, quite predictably, upon a specific face. The face for that mask belonged to someone dead. The earliest known masks, discovered near modern day Jerusalem, were fashioned to honor ancestors and provide a glimpse into some of the earliest known communal rituals as Neolithic societies were transitioning from hunter-gatherer models into stable farming groups. Because they were made of stone, they survived. They didn't have a whole lot of detail. There were likely other masks at this time fashioned from wood and leather; these would have degraded, leaving few traces. There is evidence of highly stylized masks in West Africa from around 7000 BCE with significantly greater detail cast in copper and bronze, as well as wood, textile, and pottery. They were decorated with animal material including hair, teeth, bones, and horns, as well as seashells, feathers, and agricultural products. These masks, like the earlier ones, played important roles in connecting ancestral spirits with their descendants; these ancestors served as protectors, so their favor was much prized for the success of the community. Mask makers connected this world and the next, serving as intermediaries to translate spirits into tangible form in order to seek their guidance and pay them honor.

West African wooden masks were a medium for communication with ancestors, animals, and spirits, playing a key role in Edo, Yoruba, and Igbo rituals to connect with those who came before as well as those who oversee fertility, harvest, and forest health. Oceanic, North American, and Aztec masks seemed to serve similar roles of ancestor communication, hunting guidance, and fertility rituals, with a rich variety of materials, decorative patterns, and modes of application and representation. Oceanic protective masks, which shielded the community from malevolent spirits, could be extremely large, whereas Latin American death masks were fitted to the faces of those who wore them. These ritual masks protected communities from poor harvest and starvation wrought by vengeful spirits and improper worship. Death masks served a related role, guiding spirits, keeping them safe on their journeys, and enabling them to communicate with and assist the living. They were not just representational but transformational; those who wore the masks often became those whom the masks depicted. Masks, both as generic categories and highly specific individualized representations, were tremendously powerful in life and death cycles, operating as medium, shield, and channel, both honoring and determining life and death.

Early Egyptian masks were also used by priests and leaders in fertility and agricultural rituals, often modelled after the likeness of an animal or God. These material artefacts took on tremendous power; that which represented the God—in this case the mask/priest composite—became the God. Masks connected this world and the next, and could call that next world into being in this one, providing direct access and animation to that which, without face, remained obscure. Masks, then, when worn in the right ritual context, were not just representations but manifestations that brought with them protection, power, pleasure, and, sometimes, pain. Masks were also a kind of map, guiding spirits back to their (preserved, mummified) bodies to have a permanent place to dwell. Death masks maintained the appearance of the face when the body had become unrecognizable due to the preservation process, helping to bring the spirit back to its bodily dwelling. The earliest death masks for the masses were made from wood; later adaptations included a technique known as cartonnage made by soaking papyrus or linen in plaster. This material was then molded on a wooden model and left to set. Royal masks reflected not just the faces but the status of those they represented, and were made of gold or gold leaf. Masks of all statuses were decorated and painted with jewels and ornaments, offering a glimpse into changing Egyptian fashions and makeup styles and techniques. Both representational and aspirational, funerary masks offered the dead the best version of their lives as they called the spirits home.

Which is to say: masks do indeed obscure access to the face, which, as the physiognomists would argue, thusly obscures access to the soul, to the ability to see the character that is writ upon the features of the other. But masks have also been used to ease the soul upon its journey away from the body toward to the world of the spirit. These masks were bridges, connecting this world to the next and the living to the dead in this moment of transition, both protecting the ancestors and offering protection from them. Dating back at least from 1938 BCE and seen in ancient Egypt, Cambodia, and the former Siam, funerary masks often had a cloth base that was layered with plaster or stucco and painted with the features of the deceased. The higher-ranking the person, the more elaborate the materials, with leaders, Pharaohs, and monarchs buried with silver or gold masks. These funerary masks were placed upon the faces of the dead to call forth the spirit. They were designed to honor the dead by helping their features endure even as they forced the soul to depart the body and begin the journey to the spirit world. They also provided a kind of shield for that potentially treacherous journey, scaring away those spirits who might wish this one harm. The funerary mask did not obscure the soul; it excavated it.

Does that make this funerary covering a mask for the soul? That question makes a lot of assumptions that the body and the soul are distinct or distinguishable entities, or at least that one can be covered while the other left bare. According to the basic principles of physiognomy, the face is the index to the soul: what you see on the outside reflects the invisible that lies beneath. By this logic, a face mask serves to mask the soul. But that's not usually its explicit intention, or not always (again: bug/feature). Certainly, masks that serve to conceal or protect identity may be said, according to physiognomic theory, to be designed to obscure the soul, or that which makes people the individuals that they are. It makes sense: a mask whose point is to make someone unidentifiable is serving as a shield to identity, to the self, to, some may say, the soul. But that's usually secondary to a more concrete self-obscuring service around evading detection or exposure. A funerary or death mask did specific things in the world (and other worlds). All masks do; perhaps the role of the mask is that which determines what it is.

Death masks performed labor beyond their spiritual uses. They were not static. There are death masks cast upon the faces of the deceased to preserve their features and preserve their memories. These were a kind of portrait, an effigy that lived on as people died. They did not obscure faces but saved them from obscurity: the face was gone from daily life from memory, and eventually, due to composition, from the earth. The masks lived on. They covered the features to reproduce them, not to hide them or take them to another place. There were, perhaps, traces of the soul, of the identity of the model in the mask that was left behind, but the point of these death masks was how they looked. They were not asked to usher a soul or protect it. They were for the living, not the dead. It's possible no one even asked the dead if they wanted one. (Such masks were usually reserved for the wealthy and powerful, and were a part of the way they were buried. Probably no one thought to ask, but I personally wouldn't want one made of my face. As a Jewish woman whose tradition has very strict rules around the treatment of dead bodies, I am highly unlikely to get one.)

Are death masks religious masks? Ritual ones? Is a funeral shroud a ritual mask? A religious one? Are dead bodies the space in which religion, ritual, and medicine intersect? Or perhaps it is sick bodies in which these meanings intersect: the roles masks have played in preventing and curing disease are not restricted to limiting the spread of germs or viruses. Masks have covered the faces of the Iroquois False Face Society, who were tasked with exiling the demons of disease from their villages. The people behind the masks were healers who brought together ritual and medicine through their pantomimes, violent productions that drove demons away. The Sri Lankan Sinhalese used at least nineteen unique sickness demon masks; bearing strong resemblance to dragons with bright colors and aggressive fangs, these masks were designed to scare sickness away. The Burkina Faso Plank Masks of the Bobo, Bwa, Kurumba, and Mossi people are representations of nature spirits in concrete form. They are worn during performances to facilitate communication between the living and the dead, people and nature, between this world and another. Both conduit and embodiment, these masks are worn not as an abstraction but a manifestation of that which is often ephemeral. They appear at funerals to accompany the dead on their journeys, and during initiation rites and agricultural festivals to ensure that these events proceed according in time and in sync. These masks are guides, rituals, media, and timekeepers, touching on all aspects of the life (and death) cycle. Fertility masks trouble the distinction between medical and ritual uses in similar ways. Many Indigenous people including the Iroquoi, Hopi, and Zuni nations use masks as part of harvest rituals to offer gratitude and safeguard future crops. Abundant harvests sustain life; fertility masks connect the body and the spirit. And, perhaps, the spirits.

5 PERFORMING AS PROTECTION

Ritual masks communicated with, called upon, and carried home ancestral and other spirits. Ancient theatrical masks were also media, consciously and publicly communicating character and expression while protecting a performer's face and experiences, keeping them private. The line between ritual, festive, and theatrical masks is porous and faint and easily stretched, twisted, altered, and erased. While some sacred masks belong firmly in one category and some performative masks belong firmly in another, many are used in festive and public contexts that necessarily encompass both. While theatre masks were not masquerades, the lines between ritual and performance were not always so clear cut. What can we call an exorcism that uses a mask to perform certain rituals for communal witnessing? How about when that same exorcism is performed on stage at a set time of year as part of a festival or celebration?

Early Greek masking was designed to both honor and placate notoriously fickle gods. As part of their ceremonial impersonation of Dionysus, worshippers would copy his practice of wearing goatskins and drinking wine. Those skins became masks, and masks made deities manifest. The mask-wearing worship brought the gods into being, and the wearer began to speak in their voices. These first-person moments of communication expanded into increasingly elaborate productions that fused ritual with play, worship with performance. In the giant amphitheaters of ancient Greece, masks not only provided visual messaging but helped amplify the performers' voices across the outdoor space.

Chinese theatrical masks use particular colors to code character, communicating key information at glance. Javanese and Balian dance dramas use wooden masks or *tupeng* to simultaneously entertain and protect against catastrophe. Drawing on Sanskrit, and specifically Hindu, epic stories, these performances developed into shadow plays with an unseen narrator who describes the actions of the actors sporting painted masks held in place by a mouth strap. Japanese *Noh* masks shifted from a strict religious framework to a more explicitly performative role around the mid to late Muromachi period (1392-1573); performers sought to hide their own mundane faces as they sought to communicate the profound aspects of the lived experience and explore the nature of mysterious beauty. While there were originally around 60 types of *Noh* masks and associated characters, there are now over 200 that remain in use and are produced by master mask makers of long familial lineage. These masks are deliberately neutral in expression, and allowed the performer to infuse the mask with emotion through a deep fusion in which the performer and mask united. Rather than performers transforming the mask, they became the mask. Masks, then, were not just an expression of emotion or character, but a way to call them into being. This too was great power.

We now recognize the shape of these character masks. Some of them instantiate characteristics and emotions, and some of them represent or indeed are specific roles, figures, people, or entities. Some of these are stable, categorized, even generic: a particular character mask, like Harlequin and Columbine from the Italian professional Commedia Dell'Arte originating in the sixteenth century, may always be represented the same way. These long historical traditions sometimes extend beyond masks to puppets and other media; others are connected through hints, trends, and subtle continuities that are reinforced and made clear by the dialogue and acting, bringing all aspects together to make manifest the role while obscuring the actor. A theatrical mask, human or—I'm thinking here of the transportive stage production of *The Lion King)* animal—can be said to protect the audience from seeing beyond the stage, and the actor from revealing too much of themselves. These masks work to hide or obscure that which would inspire doubt or limit immersion into the experience; they also obscure that which brings them into being. The actor as an individual, and as an actor, must be estranged or made distant from the from the role, and the mask serves to create such a distance precisely in order to bring the two together.

Theatrical masks are not just cues and representations. They are transportive media, akin in a way to the deglamming that many actors do to immerse themselves in a role, and that is a vital mechanism for iconic actors in particular. Some call it playing ugly to be taken seriously, as, say, Charlize Theron did in *Monster*, or Nicole Kidman did in *The Hours*. But it's more than that: it's a technique to separate the icon from the character, so that the audience can fully suspend disbelief and engage in the narrative. Iconicity entails in large part the impossibility of such a separation; Marilyn is always Marilyn and is always there, no matter who she is playing or how good she is at it. Deglamming serves as the mask—literal, in terms of facial prosthetics and alterations, and theoretical, in terms of the work it does—which reminds both audience and actor to try to forget. Mask here is both material and metaphor, trick and theatrical technique. Actor Oscar Isaac turned to his Juilliard training to do "mask work" for a recent Paul Schrader film. Schrader is well known for his insistence on internality and stoicism from his actors, calling upon them to be, in a way, the opposite of icons, sublimating not just their celebrity but all emotion into the narrative. Isaac understood this to mean that, as he said to the *New York Times*, "my face is going to literally be a mask," so he sought to "tell the story just through the body and through energy." Deglamming and interiority are masks in and of themselves, not just to render a well-known face unrecognizable, but to allow an icon to disappear. It may be a career risk, but it's also a kind of freedom.

6 FREEDOM AND CONSTRAINT

WHOSE TRUST MATTERS

Protecting one person may mean endangering another. Narratives of protection are often a cover for enabling other forms of oppression or endangerment, and it's usually those in power who benefit. We tell Black men to make themselves appear less threatening, which protects us from encountering our own embedded racism. We put cameras in public spaces and trade privacy for security and create systems that make many people less safe. We tell women to dress a certain way for their protection, which protects society from getting at the root of what makes women's lives and bodies subject to attack. We expose women to make sure men know exactly who and what they are getting. Metaphorically. But also in moments of sacred union.

I was at a wedding last spring at a beautiful B&B (NOT an Airbnb™, but the old fashioned kind) in the Pocono Mountains in Pennsylvania. The ceremony was in a little clearing a distance from the buildings, with a *chuppah* (Jewish wedding canopy) fashioned within a twisted tree trunk sculpture. Before the ceremony, the bride and groom held *tisches* (tables), a raucous series of short talks that are traditionally interrupted with singing and jokes. At the conclusion, the groom was danced over to the bride, where he lowered her veil, the *bedekin*, over her face. It's a lovely and romantic moment, and often the first time the couple has seen one another that day, or even over several days. (Not this couple: they were hanging out all morning.) Tears were shed. Everyone was hushed. Except me. I gasped and said: mask! The veil too, is a mask. It covers. It conceals. And, metaphorically, it protects. Sort of. Its absence protects. The moment of covering protects. And then, the face is gone.

Let me clarify. In the biblical story of Jacob and Laban, Jacob is tricked into marrying Leah when he wanted to marry her sister Rachel. Laban extorts an additional 7 years of labor from Jacob in exchange for gifting Rachel to Jacob as an additional wife. Leah's face, the commentators explain, was covered; Jacob did not know that she was not Rachel. So—at least according to Rabbinic tradition—a groom himself place the veil over his bride's face to make sure she are who she says she is. The protection then, is for the groom, from trickery, deception, concealed identity and from the veil itself—from the mask itself. It is the act of masking that offers protection that disappears in the moment the act is done. The veil carries within its biblical origins the duality of, and tensions around, protection for and protection from. According to the text, when Jacob's mother Rebecca saw her intended groom Isaac for the first time, she donned her veil, protecting her modesty and, at the same time, creating a barrier between her and her future partner.

While most veils are gauzy and translucent and really can't hide much identity at all, some do. It is a practice amongst certain ultra-Orthodox Jewish sects to add an additional piece of cloth to the veil, one that is entirely opaque. The first time I witnessed this custom was at a cousin's wedding, the second time at the wedding of a dear friend from childhood who had become much more observant after university. In both cases, the bride walked into her wedding ceremony completely unable to see. She was guided by her mother and mother-in-law, who walked her down the aisle and held her arms during the traditional seven circuits around the groom. The support these women offered was not metaphorical: the bride could see nothing and needed people to guide her. There's a lot of metaphor in that. But also: sometimes the protection afforded by a mask is the moment when it is removed. Or the moment before it is put on. Some might say we need to be protected *from* the mask. It all depends on who and how we defend. It all depends on who and how we trust.

The question of trust is very much at stake in the anti-masking laws that emerged in the United States in 1845 in response to property riots in upstate New York. These laws, which are still extant in a number of US States and various countries around the world, prohibit masking in public in order to supposedly prevent people from anonymously committing crimes because, undetectable, they would be free from the threat of prosecution and punishment. Similar justifications have been used in Quebec and France to proscribe the Muslim hijab (veil) and niqab (face covering), claiming that this kind of facial obscuring comprises a limitation of personhood, makes the wearer unidentifiable and thus a kind of (untrustworthy) security risk, and needs to be legislated against for both the good of the individual and of society.

These places don't have similar limitations on wearing warm scarves, or hockey masks, or surgical masks. What could be the difference between a niqab and an American football helmet? What could be the difference between a person protesting rental hikes and one covering his face with a white hood to participate in a lynching?

What indeed. It seems as though it's less about what the mask obscures than whom it obscures. It seems that some people have more right to mask than others. Any niqabi and any Black man in the pandemic could have told you that already. It actually *is* about trust, and the plausible deniability that the mask provides to excuse racism and Islamophobia. We aren't quite so concerned about verifying the identities of our doctors or athletes as we are about Muslim women. Could it be that it's not the hijab or niqab that's the problem, but our relationship to it?

Life doesn't always provide a case study. Rare is a naturally repeated experiment that demonstrates a particular claim. But the searing legal hypocrisy that required hijabis and niqabis in France and Quebec to remove their religious masks while donning surgical ones in public buildings could not have been laid barer. In the midst of a global health crisis, there was still space to maintain Islamophobia even while attending to collective health and safety. Early in the pandemic, France levied a 130 euro fine on those who appeared in public without their Covid masks while maintaining an even higher fine for wearing a niqab. In Quebec, Bill 21 continued to criminalize religious masking even as it required medical masking. A hospital patient would be asked to remove her niqab even as she was handed a Covid mask. It was never about being able to identify people. It was never about the threat of obscured faces. And Muslim women who veil were not surprised. Outraged, but not surprised. The motivations behind the anti-religious masking were not and had never been confusing to them.

One Canadian niqabi made her frustration clear with a wink and a (covered) smile. Early in the pandemic, Maria Iqbal wrote an article for *Chatelaine* magazine entitled "4 Tips on Wearing A COVID-19 Mask, From a Niqabi." This friendly-seeming and generous article offers several useful hints about how to be heard, protect skin, wear glasses, and, importantly, communicate emotion, while wearing a lower-face-obscuring covering. The tips are indeed valuable, and ones that quickly became second nature to the pandemic mask-wearing masses. Embedded in these cheerful guidelines is a more poignant message: what is new to you is familiar to me. What was once problematic is now quotidian. What made me stand out makes you blend in. We are all mask wearers now. (And: Was my kind of mask so very bad? *Why* was this mask so very bad?)

The tone of the piece echoes the hints Iqbal shares about how to convey feeling to others even with the (expressive) mouth obscured. Specifically, Iqbal is careful (so careful!) to emphasize, how to "exchange happy glances," how to smile with your eyes" (aka "smize," iykyk). For the already vulnerable publicly Muslim woman, it makes great sense to be careful to project friendliness and maximize anything that could contribute to being perceived as non-threatening. Her niqab is itself, for too many people, a source of threat; Iqbal does her best to negate this unfair association with her very being, in so far as she can without a visible mouth smile. She highlights here the reality of mask-aided interaction, teaching us how to over perform our eyes, emphasize our eyebrows and other visible parts of our face as indices to that which is obscured. She already knew how to do this, having spent so much time using her visible features to make others feel at ease.

Iqbal, in the framing of writer Brent Staples, is whistling Vivaldi. Staples coined this term as a description of his experience of literally whistling Vivaldi in Chicago's Hyde Park after dark. His strategy was to signal his education and refinement music in order to calm the fears of white passersby. Classical music whistlers, even those who are Black men, Staples reasoned, do not read as violent and dangerous. The logic extends well beyond Staples. In a 2020 article in *The Pigeon*, writer Leila El Shennawy discusses Covid masks with a number of niqabis; a clear theme emerges. Many of the women she talks with have long employed similar strategies to Iqbal. Some are more explicit about their motivations; Shaheen Ashraf, a Board Member of the Canadian Council of Muslim women, has become accustomed to working hard to put those around her at ease. In the article, Ashraf said that people were very nervous around her after 9/11, so she deliberately offered compliments to those around her, including telling someone in the elevator, "that's a nice handbag. Where did you get it?" The response was immediate and Ashraf "could literally feel the fear melt away. Like 'Phew, she's normal.'" Quebec high school teacher Nadia Naqvi had a visceral reaction to being in public, telling a friend that she was "kind of scared of going to Walmart." Her friend urged her to, simply, "try just smiling." Naqvi tried smiling. She had "this dumb half smile on my face" and learned that "people respond to that." "That," of course, being the smile that others couldn't even see. That smile, of course, being the "dumb half" variant. Dumb because forced. Half because defensive. Necessary because niqab.

Anti-niqab rhetoric is rooted in this idea that people who can't be identified represent a security risk. (That doesn't explain why "burkinis" or full-body coverage bathing suits, are banned in public pools in France. Nor does the stated explanation of hygiene, which isn't an explanation at all. Surely full-body and -hair coverage is more hygienic?) Some people wear masks only when they are about to engage in activities for which they do not want to be identified and detected. On some level, this narrative makes a kind of sense: if you are in a bank and someone comes in wearing a stocking on their face, you probably want to get out as fast as possible. But surely, as we do with athletes, cold people, and health care practitioners, we can tell the difference between one kind of masking and another.

As we have seen by the general lack of concern around needing to identify people who wear Covid masks, context matters. I live in South Philadelphia. The hijab is a common sight, and local African American Muslim women wear a version of niqab and abaya. Growing up in a heavily Jewish neighborhood in Toronto, seeing niqabis was, for me, rather rare. My associations with religious head covering and modesty rules were exclusively Jewish: some women followed the custom of covering their hair after marriage with hats, or kerchiefs, or (fewer, in my experience, but some were so sophisticated I couldn't tell) *sheitels* or wigs. And of course, many boys and men, including those in my school, wore *kippot*, or yarmulkes on their heads. These are not masks, though sheitels may be masks for hair. I'd seen niqabs in the airport and trips outside my neighborhood, and, when I was 17, on my summer teen tour to Israel. Toronto is a heavily multicultural city, and once I was old enough to venture outside of my enclave, I encountered and learned about a lot of communities. I certainly saw hijabs, and Sikh turbans and Amish bonnets. By the time I got to university I had exposure to a wide range of religious garments and traditions. But my most enduring memory of these forms of Muslim modesty clothing remained, for a long time, a 2002 episode of the television show JAG entitled "Head to Toe."

I wasn't a regular watcher of JAG (or, at that point in my life, any particular television show with the exception of *Buffy the Vampire Slayer* which played in reruns at 7 am when I went to the gym) but happened to catch this episode when I was at home visiting my family. It stuck with me, less because of the central conflict than the reaction of the JAGs—the naval lawyers assigned to prosecute and defend those in the service in naval court—to the female pilot they were assigned to defend. The main characters, Harm and Mac, had to fly to Saudi Arabia to defend a naval pilot who publicly refused to comply with the requirement to wear an abaya and veil in public. These strictures were in place when she was engaging in food drops and other operational activities. The pilot, Lieutenant Joanne Donato, also drove herself rather than sitting in the back of a car chauffeured by a male escort as was required of women in Saudi Arabia at the time. Mac (played by Catherine Bell) was initially frustrated with Donato's seeming insubordination; soldiers do as they are told. (I remembered none of this, for the record, but everything is available for a rewatch these days.) I *do* remember, in clear detail and twenty years on, the moment when Mac changed her mind. Forced herself to abide by these policies, Mac experienced the difference between thinking and embodying, seeing and doing. It wasn't just how she felt under clothing cover and with only her eyes visible—it was how others treated her. She was knocked over, ignored, and lost her individuality, status, and public identity. She—and other military women—could not be saluted appropriately by subordinates as their rank and identity were unknown.

The episode was meant to raise questions about the balance between respecting local cultures and customs and insisting on maintaining one's own sense of human rights and justice. It's also a show about the military, and, inevitably, about conquest and violence and imperialism (dressed up in navy whites with David James Elliot's winning smile and inexhaustible charm.) The US military has a mission, and any showcase of the institution is part of that mission. (What's the pithy term for the military version of copaganda?) It also viscerally communicates the very real stakes for forcing women to adhere to a particular set of clothing norms. Mac was responding to an erasure engendered by covering her body and face. The episode supports this narrative, underscoring the challenges the abaya and driving restrictions posed to both Donato and Mac in being able to effectively do their jobs (as members of the US navy in a foreign country). Donato was, we see, frequently harassed in public, shamed, and mocked for her dress. Mac was assaulted and ignored. Perhaps it was the clothing. Perhaps it was a broader misogyny. It's fiction, though certainly not fantasy. But Mac may also have been responding to having these conditions forced upon her. She knew the rules that all women, including Donato, were required to follow in Saudi Arabia, and she, as a member of the military, supported rules and the necessity of following them. But there is a difference between knowing and feeling. When she had to experience these rules, she felt why they were unjust. And she felt keenly the conflict between the obligations of her role in the navy and the following of these particular rules. The navy obligations superseded, for her, the laws of a land that was not her own.

Had the rules been in consonance, had she not felt her ability to do her job undermined by these restrictions, would Mac or Donato have objected with quite the same fervor? Would the lived experience of having their fundamental dignity and human rights undermined have been enough to object to this practice with which they did not agree? Was it the forcing, or the fact of what was being forced, which felt to Mac much worse in practice than in theory? It's fiction and I can't answer these questions. But in presenting the Islamophobia inherent in hijab and niqab bans on the one hand, and the misogyny of punitively forcing certain clothing on women on the other, I wish to emphasize that both cases undermine women's choice and agency, and that in neither case is trusting those whose agency is robbed really at stake.

Only a minority of Muslim women choose to wear the niqab, though perhaps unsurprisingly more began to don this form of cover during the pandemic. Amid the raging intolerance and weaponization of facial covering that we saw in many parts of the world and especially the US space was opened for some Muslim women to feel newly comfortable covering their faces. Public face covering became a newly legible category. For some Muslim women, the choice was about safety to explore this form of observance; for others, there was an imperative to clarify that their masking practice was not just a public health commitment but a religious one. While many of these women also wore masks beneath their niqab or fashioned their niqab to be effective public health masks, they wanted their identity as niqabis to be clear. Also clear? It's not *that* people cover their faces that raises concern. It's who.

7 MEDICAL MASKS AND THE COVID ELEPHANT

It isn't only niqabis who have to navigate the fraught and dangerous challenges posed by publicly exposed racism and violence. Early in the pandemic, Black men did a lot of mask-related Vivaldi whistling. Black men in the US have always done a lot of prophylactic Vivaldi whistling to make those around them comfortable, to emphasize that they have a right to occupy communal space, to make it clear that they belong and do not pose a threat. Black men and women have had to avoid arousing the suspicions of those around them simply for being Black in public. In racist America in the twenty-first century (and the twentieth, and the nineteenth), being Black in public can be fraught with danger because of the danger people imagine Blackness poses. A Black man with his face covered, even when legally mandated due to Covid, is even more threatening. As sociologist Rashawn Ray catalogued, many Black families specifically chose bright masks with cheerful themes, smiles, or messages printed on them precisely to avoid arousing the racist fear of those around them. These "cheerful" Vivaldi masks were a signaling mechanism, an extension of self: not just the selves of the wearers but the society they inhabit. Masks, and also mirrors. Necessary on multiple levels of lifesaving. Black men, despite the mandates to the contrary and no matter how loudly they whistled, were still often asked to remove their masks.

Our associations with masks have changed rather dramatically during the pandemic. In the early days, a lack of PPE (personal protective equipment) had many scrambling to dig up old masks left behind during home renovation projects or unexpected fumigation events. I happened to find three masks left over from when we did our basement in 2011. A friend of mine who works in the court system and whose husband is a cardiac surgeon were both still going in to work in April 2020 and gratefully picked them up. They were better than nothing.

We all pulled out our sewing machines. We all became crafters. We all started baking bread and talking about our sourdough starters and sewing curtains and building furniture, but first, we made masks. We downloaded instructions and dug out old bandannas and some of us even learned the "make a mask out of a t-shirt without even sewing" method. There were all kinds of generous souls devoting their time to making masks and sending them to anyone who asked for free, for the cost of shipping, for a slight donation. These were masks born of fear, and boredom, and lags in the global supply chain. These were masks of solidarity and ignorance and immediate response. These weren't very good masks. They were the best we had. They were the best we—the overwhelming majority of us who were not the emergency planning infrastructure—could do. It wasn't great. That infrastructure's best, it turned out, was also not great. It was actually pretty terrible. There should and could have been better masks available, and it shouldn't have been up to The Gap to supply them.

These early pandemic masks were, of course, about protection: from the virus, from one another, from our own fear and confusion. And they were about solidarity and communality: we were, no matter how poor our crafting skills or how ugly our old t-shirts, in this together. These masks, not yet weaponized, not yet commercialized, not yet all that effective, still worked. Maybe not so much at preventing the spread of Covid-19 (though they were certainly much, much better than the nothing that was to come, and the nothing that many, even then, wore), but at making people feel like they were in control of something, anything, when so much was out of control. And they worked at making people feel connected to one another. The circulation and sharing of mask making, as much as the publicity of mask wearing, worked at uniting an always-and-soon-to-be-again fractured populace in a common goal: the elimination of a deadly virus and the reestablishment of normal life.

(This is a utopian vision. Many in the US and globally did not participate for a variety of reasons, which significantly lowered the effectiveness of mask wearing. Utopias are rhetoric-rich places.)

The early pandemic mask, usually cloth, often hand-sewn, sometimes fashionable, meant many things. It was about epidemiological logics, it was about communal norms, and it was about identity. It was about who believed in science and who believed in pandemic responses and who believed in protecting others alongside themselves. It was about boredom and generosity and desperation and longing. These masks were an extension of belief whose very presence meant something about the wearer.

The bias against masking got really confusing during the pandemic. Which form of protection do we value more highly—that which protects us against encountering our own biases, or that which protects us from disease? You'd think it would have been obvious. It was not. That, opaquely, is a statement about race, a noticing that early in the pandemic Black men sometimes found themselves asked to remove their masks despite local public health ordinances. Some people were more afraid of Black men in masks then the pandemic itself. (These may have been the same people who weren't concerned about the pandemic, or public health, or the lives of others, those who resisted masks for a variety of reasons. There are some obvious points of overlap.)

And then, on May 25, 2020, George Floyd was murdered in Minneapolis by Officer Derek Chauvin. The rhetoric around necessity and urgency changed. People took to the streets to protest yet another murder of a Black man. But it was still a pandemic, and the Black community in particular was still being hit hard by Covid. It was still early in our pandemic journey, and we didn't know that being outside was probably a lot safer than it felt. People took the streets in protest, and most people wore masks. Those masks became an extension of identity in new ways, a mirror of a different part of our social reality. We began to see masks with political slogans, messages, and protests. It was not just wearing the mask itself that said something about the person wearing it—the mask was also a message.

It was a brief moment, before we (as a world) switched pretty much exclusively to disposable masks, and while we (or some of us) were still vigilantly masking outside with less effective masks. We were doing the best we could in an evolving situation with imperfect information. Many people who wanted to join the national protests against police violence in spring of 2020 were also wary of large gatherings and concerned about public health. As a result, those marches were typically well-spaced and carefully organized, with ample room between participants. And most were wearing masks, some of the plain or homemade or fashion or—a minority—disposable variety. They probably grabbed them from the suddenly ubiquitous mask basket by the front door as they headed out. (If they were vigilant, they put them in the wash, or in the "dirty mask basket" when they got home. I'll be honest: I didn't always do that right away.)

Marching in support of racial justice was a message. Wearing masks while marching was—perhaps surprisingly, given what we thought we knew about Covid and how to stop it, given that most people don't actually want to contract a potentially deadly and certainly potentially debilitating disease—a message. And soon, inevitably, the masks themselves bore political, social, and cultural slogans. We figured out a new way for masks to serve as an extension of self, a way to express on the surface that which lay beneath. We used masks as a slate upon which to self-consciously and deliberately reveal ourselves and our messages, even as, and perhaps in response or solution to, its work to conceal. Masks became medium and message, bearing slogans subversion and positions and provocations. (My favorite may be the B"H/ Biden-Harris masks, bearing the Jewish acronym for *baruch hashem*, "may the divine name be blessed.") Handmade or mass-produced, the message mask introduced a new kind of physiognomy onto the face it covered.

Naomi Osaka's 2020 US Tennis Open run showcased message masking on center court. For each of her matches, Osaka wore a different mask bearing the name of a Black person who died from police and/or racial violence. Even given her unbeaten path to the finals during which she wore a mask with the name of twelve-year old police murder victim Tamir Rice, that was only seven masks. She could have made far, far more. Osaka, a woman of color in a historically white sport, was doing the opposite of whistling Vivaldi. She wanted to make people uncomfortable—not with her, but with the deadly system of violence and discrimination. She wanted to make people uncomfortable with our complacency within that system. Tennis matches are notoriously quiet relative to other public athletic games; Osaka found a way to scream.

As mask ordinances emerged across the US and the world, so too did mask protestors, turning to the very same autonomy and freedom of speech and body claims that motivated opposition to anti-mask laws. When forced to wear masks, many of these protestors either wore them ineffectively or offered their own slogans and political messages. There is a good-faith version of these protests; bodily autonomy and the right to abortion in particular is both a fundamental right and deeply under threat in the US at this very moment. Most of the protests against masking were not in good faith. Mask ordinances were a temporary injunction designed to support public health in public spaces. Individual rights do not extend to causing harm to autonomous others. As the refusal of the mask became weaponized as a tool of political dissent, its lack was a weapon in a more literal way as Covid continued to spread. Virulently, as, of course, it would.

Recent studies have emerged casting doubt on the efficacy of mask wearing as it was enacted and executed in the US and globally. And, of course, even more recent responses have pointed out the various and complicated ways those data could be (mis)interpreted. Here, I point out that masking remains, to the best of our knowledge, an important, affordable, and accessible technology of medical protection to limit transmission of airborne viruses. And I'll point out that this technology of protection revealed (again) the depths of discrimination and the shallowness of narratives of trust as Black men were still asked to remove their (often cheerful, brightly colored) masks. In those early days of the pandemic, racism, it turned out, trumped (Trumped?) public health. Some people deserved protection, and others, it seemed, we needed protecting from. Except that of course we all needed to protect others from each of us, and we needed to do it together, or it wouldn't work nearly as well. Which meant that everyone's faces had to be concealed, and our reactions to that—asking some people to remove their masks, using masks for political messaging and other slogans, mask refusal—revealed a whole lot. We can see a lot about people when their faces are covered.

8 VIOLENCE AND THE MASKS OF WAR

Theatrical masks, religious masks, transplanted faces as masks, the intricate and loving and complicated masks that American sculptor Anna Coleman Ladd and British artist Francis Derwent Wood made for disfigured soldiers after the First World War: these masks were not primarily or at least not exclusively about prevention. These were masks that gave rather than took, that enhanced and heighten rather than limited and obscured. They communicated emotion; they extended identity; they emphasized clarity and meaning. For the facially disfigured, these masks, along with the plastic surgery innovations of surgeon Harold Delf Gilles, allowed returning injured soldiers to navigate public space. They allowed the wearers to create connections with others that would otherwise be hard to reach, invisible, impossible, ignoring and ignored. And they allowed others to not have to interrogate their discomfort with looking injury in the face.

These are masks that emerged from violence, a way to suture the crisis of the visibly injured solider returning home. It's much harder to engage in an orgy of nationalistic triumphalism when your discomfort and ableism prevents you from treating those who achieved it as fully human. That's a different kind of protection: for society, from facing its own biases, from facing those who bore the brunt of war; but also protection for the soldiers from seeing the disgust in others, from navigating life with the eyes of others averted.

The gas mask is a curious artifact of technology, originally designed to protect the wearer from inhaling dangerous chemicals or particles. First used by minors in the late eighteenth century, early breathing devices acted as filters; by the early twentieth century, they became respirators with their own air supply, enabling longer wear and a more robust defense against potential chemical damage. These were niche items designed for those at greatest risk. And then the risk itself became ever greater with the introduction of chemical warfare in the First World War. Germans first introduced poison gas at the second battle of Ypres with devastating effects for both sides. The diffusion of the gas was difficult to control. The Allies first responded by issuing muslin-wrapped cotton wool to serve as a filter, later developing mass-produced respirators that grew in sophistication alongside the chemical warfare itself. Initially distributed only amongst those on the front lines, gas masks later became a symbol of total war, with young children during the Cold War practicing gas mask drills in schools, sometimes wearing them for an entire day to acclimate to the discomfort. The gas mask represents some of the most horrific impulses of violence and war, the last defense against a weapon whose targets cannot be entirely controlled or contained, sometimes by design. The protection afforded by a gas mask is of the most basic bodily sort, attempting to keep combatants and non-combatants— young and old, healthy and ill—undamaged, or at the very least alive. The gas mask is designed to protect individuals from the ravages of chemical and, increasingly, biological warfare, preventing further spread of disease agents but not stopping the initial infection. The gas mask does not protect societies from developing ever more dangerous ways to circumvent it. The global weapons industry continues to hide behind this inadequate form of protection in pursuit of ever greater forms of destruction.

9 NO WAY TO HIDE

The mask, according to a particular surveillance rhetoric in our increasingly surveilled world, obscures access to identification. This narrative pits security against privacy in ways that make sense in some contexts—as I said, I too would be concerned if someone came into a bank with a stocking over their face—and makes no sense in others—as we saw with the niqab. The trade-off between privacy and security manifests in multiple contexts that are at least somewhat contingent on being able to track people.

It's a trade-off that, for a long time, didn't really work all that well. Face recognition technology didn't, for a long time, work well. There are all kinds of reasons for this failure: false positives that happened because there was a limited number of women and people of color in the starting database, meaning that they were far more likely to be incorrectly identified as a match; technical limitations on what could be captured by the cameras; and, of course, people's ability to evade detection by covering their features, which is what the system relies on to determine if someone is a match for a given person of interest. I could go into a lot more depth here (and I do elsewhere, as do the wonderful scholars Nikki Stevens and Os Keyes, among others) but the key point is that face masks of all sorts were a pretty effective way to befuddle covert systems of surveillance, something which people seeking to do precisely this were completely aware of.

These systems work by turning the face into a series of unique measurements that are then compared to the measurement of faces already in the database (which is practically everyone, at this point). The algorithms needed more data points than a covered face would provide. It wasn't that the systems needed full faces to create a robust comparison; rather, they needed to be able to convert features and their relative distances to the sets of numbers that would serve as identifiers. It's a math problem, not an image problem. And now, given how rich the starting database is, how sophisticated the capture mechanisms are, and the extent to which systems can map 3D extensions of the face from just a small amount of 2D data, masks and even plastic surgery aren't always enough to evade detection.

Plastic surgery, digital filters and IRL fillers, image manipulators, and even makeup are all a form of masking, some temporary, some more permanent, some irrevocable. People manipulate their appearance for all kinds of reasons that have nothing to do with evading surveillance, and we'll discuss these interventions and their relationship to masking later. But some people do in fact change their appearance in order not to be recognized by various systems of surveillance, criminal justice, and law enforcement. Sometimes, as we've already established, it's a simple as a stocking cap over the head that makes someone unrecognizable when committing a crime or act of civil disobedience, or when engaging in terror and racist violence. (And yes, even that is nuanced: the anonymity is partly about escaping consequences from structures of law and civil society, and partly about escaping consequences from one's own identity and sense of self.) Sometimes the evasion has to last a lot longer than a singular event, and a removable face cover just won't cut it. So, cutting does.

Plastic surgery in this context is a very specific type of mask, sharing more with bandanas than blush, an attempt to fundamentally change appearance rather than to enhance it. Famous fugitives from British train robber Ronnie Biggs (1829-2013) to Columbia drug kingpin Juan Carlos Ramírez Abadía (b. 1963) famously operated on their faces as part of their attempts to avoid prosecution for their crimes. Abadía, by his own testimony (when he was eventually caught, and only due to wiretapping because he was unrecognizable facially) had multiple procedures, and, it seemed, grew to like the process. But there is no doubt that their initial surgeries were a very specific kind of mask designed to obscure their features and render themselves unrecognizable.

Plastic surgery has certainly gotten more sophisticated over time; facial recognition software even more so. Aside from a few specific procedures that change the underlying bones and thus facial structure, no single intervention will do it on its own. The algorithms can extract enough unique data from even a single feature, meaning that even with masks covering the face, and even with plastic surgery, enough of our faces remain visible and identifiable. Surveillance is just that good. And just that bad, if you value your privacy even if you aren't a fugitive, if you happen to live in an oppressive regime, or if you would like to engage in an act of protest or civil disobedience. There are endless YouTube and TikTok tutorials on how to apply "dazzle camouflage" or other forms of makeup to befuddle the technology. Spoiler alert: they mostly don't work. Your best bet is to cover your face entirely, and absolutely do not forget to obscure your ears, which are an easily accessed and highly unique feature, or, to the tech, set of data points.

The Guy Fawkes/Anonymous mask offered rather comprehensive facial coverage, becoming both symbol of protest and enabler of it. Based on a stylized depiction of seventeenth-century participant in the failed English gunpowder plot to assassinate King James I, the mask was deployed in the graphic novel *V for Vendetta*. Following the film adaptation in 2005, the hacktivist group Anonymous adopted the mask, as did those engaging in public protest. A character in its own right, the mask provided communal anonymity and practical protection from surveillance and prosecution.

Once upon a time, a global pandemic in which most people wore masks would have been a problem for surveillance structures. Not anymore. Well, unless the surveillance structure is the vast majority of people working at the Transportation Security Administration. With or without masks, when it comes to matching people to their passport photos, they tend to be right only between seventy and eighty percent of the time, which means they are wrong a whole lot, no masks necessary. (Super recognizers are right much more of the time, but most of them are not TSA agents, and most TSA agents are not super recognizers.)

The rhetoric around religious masking was always hypocritical and contingent upon the *who* rather than the *what*. I do not wish to minimize the very powerful effects of seeing others face-to-face and how that helps build relationships and create recognition and affinity. There are of course other ways to forge these connections that do not violate religious commitment and autonomy. And also, from the perspective of oppressive systems of surveillance, the notion of removing religious masks as a means of safety and trust simply does not make sense, rotted as it is in colonialist frameworks of who is valuable and trustworthy.

While facial recognition technology can identify even people wearing masks, many of us cannot. Or not easily, and certainly with heavy reliance on other clues including voice, gait, hair, clothing styles, and context. It is much more complicated for people to know who others are at a glance when their noses and mouths are obscured. How can we tell who the heroes and villains are anymore? (Spoiler alert: we never reliably could.)

10 VILLAIN/HERO

V'NAHAFOCH HU

I want to return to trust, trustworthiness, and to the mask as obstructive and revelatory.

Let's switch it up.

The use of "switch" is a bit of insider baseball. It's a reference to the Jewish holiday of Purim, a strange and fairly subversive festival that involves subterfuge, assassination attempts, deliberately intoxicating an enemy, a false sexual assault scenario, a strategic intermarriage between a (possibly already betrothed) Jewish woman and the monarch, and a massive (murderous) party.

Briefly: the scene is ancient Persia. The monarch is a drunken libertine called Achashverosh. He banishes (or perhaps executes) his primary wife, Vashti, after she refuses to appear naked at one of his parties. The search for a new primary wife is launched, and all young maidens, including a young Jewish woman named Esther, are prepped for their auditions. (While this is an extra-textual reading, the custom of the time was that those not selected as chief partner after their sexual audition would, as defiled maidens, join the King's harem as concubines. The stakes were high.) Esther is chosen. Under the guidance of her relative (and possible betrothed) Mordechai, she hides her Jewish identity. A good thing, too, because Achashverosh's advisor and egomaniac-in-chief, Haman (*yimach shemo*), takes against the Jews after Mordechai refused to follow the dictum to bow to Haman in the public square. Haman convinces the king to issue a decree calling for the slaughter of the Jewish people on a day selected by *pur*, or lottery (thus the name). Esther, in a cunning series of parties, saves the day. The decree is countered, allowing the Jews of the realm to defend themselves. Celebrations ensue. Along the way, there are assassination attempts, hangings, and various other shenanigans. To mark the deferral of genocide, Jewish communities engage in a number of ritual revelries, including a celebratory meal, sending baskets of treats, hearing the *megillah* (the scroll that recounts the story), and, indeed, wearing costumes and masks. (And alcohol. In some communities, lots and lots of alcohol. Or at least enough, as per Rabbinic tradition, for revelers to be unable to distinguish between the supposed hero, Mordechai, and the clear villain, Haman. Alcohol, and subsequent inebriation from it, is also a kind of mask. And a kind of revelation.)

Purim is a holiday of revelation. It's a moment of concealing and then revealing the truth of one's identity and humanity: Esther hides her Jewishness, and then, for the sake of her people and at great personal risk, exposes it. Haman poses as a wise councilor, and, with the help of Esther (and, notably, the only vaguely framed "someplace else," the one possible and even then questionable reference to the divine) and a fateful slip, his true calculating nature emerges. It's a story of inversion, of flipping, of hiding and showing. Even the name, *Megillat Esther* (the scroll of Esther) is a cognate of *legalot hester,* to reveal the hidden.

And to honor and mark this holiday of revelation, Jewish communities around the world wear masks? It's a curious way to emphasize exposure. It's a curious way to emphasize what it means to be seen.

There is, of course, a narrative. (When it comes to Jewish tradition and practice, there are several centuries worth of narrative.) The starting point is inversion: this is an upside-down world where our assumptions are challenged and our pieties are laid bare. V'nahafoch hu. It's a story unlike other classical Jewish texts; at its heart is an intermarriage based on a subterfuge, and its conclusion is days of merry slaughter. The masks suggest that by covering our faces and our lives, we reveal the realities of all that lie beneath. That's aphoristic and vague. More specifically, the holiday highlights the ways that we live our lives behind a (sorry) metaphoric mask; on Purim, we deliberately and mindfully don masks to expose our true selves.

The Twilight Zone often made the metaphorical literal. In a 1964 episode entitled "The Masks," a dying patriarch prepared a surprise for his terrible offspring who reluctantly visited him in New Orleans on the eve of Mardi Gras. There only for his fortune, his daughter, her husband, and their two children were annoyed at having to visit him in his last moments. As a final condition of their inheritance, the patriarch insisted they each wear a carefully crafted Cajun mask, which, "in addition to their artistic value," "have certain properties." Each mask reflected the true character of the wearer, despite their own self-assessment to the contrary. Although, in the patriarch's words, "one tries to select a mask that is the antithesis of what the wearer is," these horrible face coverings rang true, representing greed, cruelty, avarice, duplicity, self-obsession, and myriad other characteristics. The faces of his family were physiognomically false, failing to represent their true caricatures. The masks rang true, and, after that fateful hour, while the physical masks could be removed, they remained imprinted, permanently altering the faces beneath. Their original faces were the masks; their masks revealed who they really were, thus wearing "the faces of all that is inside them."

If this plot sounds cinematically familiar, it's because it is. We've discussed here the deep roots of masks calling characters into being in ritual and performative contexts across cultures, and we've seen how these themes manifest in the Purim story and celebration. *The Twilight Zone* offers us one version of not just the revelatory but transformative powers of the mask, bringing character to the surface and inscribing it on the face forever. The 1966 Japanese film *The Face of Another* directed by Hiroshi Teshigahara features a prosthetic mask that causes the wearer to act in dramatically different ways. Based on a 1964 novel by Kōbō Abe, the film highlights how a mask creates new possibilities for behavior and the public self. The story is deliberately ambiguous about if the mask excavates and provides the conditions of possibility for someone to be who they always were, or if it is the primary agent of change in the wearer. The face is of another person: the new face may have created him or it may have enabled him to finally be himself. The mask in the film resonates with the fantasy masks in the 1926 Teinosuke Kinugasa silent film *A Page of Madness*. The protagonist dreams of distributing happy faced-masks to the inmates of the asylum in which he works as a janitor partly to be closer to his inmate wife, hoping to excavate or transform their way of being in the world and turn madness into joy. The face-as-mask contains great revelatory, or perhaps transformative, power.

In *The Mask* (1994), a nebbish wallflower named Stanley Ipkiss has his life changed by his discovery of a wooden green mask. When Ipkiss puts it on, he becomes a mischievous superhero who wreaks all kinds of havoc and puts Stanley and those around him in danger. The mask was created by the Norse god of mischief Loki; when Ipkiss puts it on, it unleashes his own deeply repressed wishes and character. The mask is the medium by which Ipkiss's desires are excavated, and it gives him the power to experience a new version of himself. This mask also reveals as it conceals, but it also causes change in Ipkiss and, correspondingly, in the world. Ipkiss's mask, unlike those of *The Twilight Zone*, can be removed, but Ipkiss himself is changed forever, becoming a fusion of who he wished he could be and who he always already was. It's a very particular kind of makeover, where a mask brings a powerful entity into being. Without the mask, Ipkiss would always only be Ipkiss. With the mask, he actually *is* The Mask, and perhaps always will be: we do not know what it leaves behind when it is finally removed,.

Sometimes we need masks to escape ourselves, and sometimes we need masks to try on another version of ourselves, and sometimes masks can do both, giving us license to experiment personally and collectively. The grotesque and exaggerated horror masks of Halloween and masquerades like Mardi Gras have served to offer communal release, license for play and experimentation, and opportunities for collective, if momentary, permission to do that which is only possible with the promise of anonymity. It's a moment of consensual disguise enabling performative and bounded transgressions whose tacit rules are known and largely respected. The mask, with its symbolic anonymity, provides the conditions of possibility for temporary release, what the literary theorist Mikhail Bakhtin called "the carnivalesque," a sensuous subversion of boundaries that celebrates the visceral, the fleshy, the physical. This celebration strips pieties bare in a profound creative collectivity that is fundamental to the human experience. In the case of Mardi Gras, that moment girds and perhaps even sustains the community for the Lenten month of deprivation and self-control, offering a particular kind of individual and group preparation for the demands ahead. The local masquerade ball serves similar ends, offering pockets of controlled release that sit alongside the rules governing polite society and social interaction when identities are undeniably known.

Stanley Kubrick's final (and not very good) film, *Eyes Wide Shut* (1999), uses masking and masquerade as a central motif, chronicling the protagonist's attempt to satisfy his wife sexually by finding and excavating another side of himself. It sort of works, and masks sort of help. Drawing on the association between masks and licentiousness, the film follows Dr. William Harford's encounter with a masquerade orgy, attempting to embrace another way of being but discovering that he has opened himself up to great danger. He can, in the end, only be who he is, but the experiment alone serves its goal, exciting his wife despite (or perhaps because of) the horrors he witnessed and describes to her. Harford's visit to the orgy is both enabled and endangered by the mask that did not entirely serve to protect him: he is publicly unmasked and his identity is easily discovered. The masks in the film literally conceal and reveal, exposing the limits to anonymity as a mode of transformation. These masks, easily and dangerously removed, highlight that people don't really change all that much; that which is done under cover is a true reflection of who they are, not who they wish to become. Masks are a gateway to both fantasy and nightmare, emphasizing that for Harford's wife, the story of the experience is all that matters. The mask helped her locate her excitement and desire by changing her perception of her husband rather than causing him to change himself.

Masks can serve as a device to upend our expectations about who people are: literally, in the sense that masks can obscure identification while leaving space to fantasize or fill in (often tantalizingly, often inaccurately) what lies beneath; and metaphorically by giving maskers plausible deniability, or license, or freedom to behave in uncharacteristic ways. (Not quite a metaphor, actually, but not quite not one.) There's historical precedent: masking was quite the trend for upper-class ladies in Europe in the early modern era.

Braden Phillips has written extensively about European masking culture in the sixteenth through eighteenth centuries for *National Geographic* magazine. Women wore masks to the theatre and in other bawdy settings as a way to protect both their social standing (by being unidentifiable) and their virtue (by making their expressions unreadable.) The vogue of masks also afforded European noblewomen a bit of freedom, allowing them to venture to spaces outside their social class under the cover of anonymity. Women developed rituals of play and seduction, particularly in seventeenth-century Paris, where they would use masks to signal interest, desire, flirtation, and (sometimes) retreat. By the middle of the eighteenth century, Parisian women were bored of masks, and found other, more casual ways to mark (modestly) rising freedom. At the same time Venice was known as the city of masks, with an almost obsessive interest in defining and policing when and how they were worn from the seventeenth through the nineteenth centuries. What began as a Carnival accessory soon spread across the year for both men and women, giving the elites greater mobility to engage with people outside their class in coffeehouses, theatres, parks, and markets.

But there was a limit to this mobility. Of course there was. Of course, the sixteenth-century "vizard," which covered the entire face and was particularly helpful in concealing the identities of women who were in places they (according to the social mores of the time) did not belong, became a slang term for prostitute. Of course, women who stretched the boundaries of their expected behavior were punished for it. And, of course, this happened in England. In 1704, Queen Anne banned vizards in theatres, removing this point of access and mode of protection for aristocratic women. But it wasn't only the elites who were affected: seventeenth-century Venetian prostitutes were also forbidden from wearing masks while plying their trade in case they were mistaken for virtuous or honest women. If this seems a bit counter-intuitive, it is: recognizing the potential of masks to serve as public markers, in the early eighteenth century the Venetian government changed course entirely, requiring all sex workers to publicly wear masks in gambling halls and theatres. But this too provided space for anonymity and a kind of dangerous (liberating?) social exchange. So, in 1776, the pendulum swung again with a decree that all nobles wear masks in pursuit of greater modesty, and perhaps to limit the opportunities granted by public anonymity or lack of accountability. There were no more mask decrees from Venice, but I'm not sure that last one worked very well.

Behind the masks, the commoner, the prostitute, and the noblewoman may all have been different; in the eyes of the crowd, they looked exactly the same. Were they so different? Their circumstances were. But usually such sentences read something like, "Beneath their skin, their beating hearts were just the same." Or, "If you prick us, do we not bleed?" Usually, it is the faces we present to the world that are seen as the markers of distinction amongst our common humanity. But this anecdote reveals that the narrative of our common humanity is a myth. We have always assigned more value to some kinds of humans over others, even though the heart of the noblewoman and the peasant both pump blood through a system and that very blood will indeed bleed. Masks make a lie of difference. Masks reveal through concealing. V'nahafoch hu. But masks can be taken off. And noblewomen go home to their gilded cages at the end of the night. Masked, they could act as they wished to. They could act as they really were. In this approach, a mask is a technology of liberation; hide your face to show your soul. Or, as in the Covid mask debates, choosing to mask is itself a way to reveal what you care about, who you care about. who you are.

That's one option. V'nahafoch hu. Let's invert it. The story of Purim is not just the story of revealing by concealing, but of concealing by revealing. The face we present to the world is not always who we actually are. Haman hid behind his position. Esther hid behind hers. And the world did not know them. Their lovers, even, did not know them. And what they chose to hide was itself a form of exposure. Maybe we don't need alcohol to confuse Haman and Mordechai because it was clear all along. Maybe Mordechai isn't really a hero. Maybe no one is the hero in a story that ends with 3 days of murder and revelry. Maybe victorious mass slaughter and self-defense isn't a cause for celebration. Maybe masks not only conceal and reveal but help us see things in a new way. Maybe the inversion here is that no one wins when people lie, cheat, hide, and hunt others.

Maybe when it comes to villains, we have it all wrong. Killmonger was a goddamn hero.

11 SUPERHEROES, OR WHO WATCHES THE WATCHERS

This isn't a book about the Marvel Cinematic Universe, or superheroes at all. But a lot of comics and superhero narratives do spend time interrogating not just masks, but how they relate to identity, power, self-awareness, and the ability to hide in plain sight. The superhero and archvillain archetypes often depend on masking as a way to exert power in public while preserving the ability to be private. *Black Panther* (2018) is a modern example of v'nahafoch hu. The titular character and leader of the secretly ultra-prosperous African nation Wakanda is by definition the hero; when challenger Killmonger, raised in the US and witness to its racism, deep structural oppression, and endemic and growing inequality, makes a run for throne, he's vying for superhero status, even though his very quest—against the good guy—means that he must be the villain. But Killmonger the villain is advocating against Wakanda's isolationist stance. He saw the wealth and privilege of this successful and secret and shuttered African country and ached, *ached*, to see it deployed to help other Black communities in desperate need. Maybe there are no villains here except the systems that exacerbate inequalities. And that includes the wildly wealthy society that largely cared only for a very narrow definition of its own. Killmonger and a lot of other people had to die for Wakanda to change its mind and lift its country-concealing, if not face-covering, mask, and reveal and share its plenty with the world. Sometimes we hide to protect ourselves from those outside. Sometimes—especially when we have the power— that's the wrong decision. But power is a tricky thing, and it's not always easy to tell who has it, especially when one feels vulnerable. Especially when there is a deep and traumatizing history of vulnerability. The line between hero and villain is not always clear.

Which brings me to the question: Who watches the watchers, especially when the watchers are themselves unseen? To put it another way: it's not just the good guys who wear masks. But didn't we know that already? Isn't that exactly why there have been anti-mask laws? I certainly wasn't confused that the Ku Klux Klan were the bad guys. But this is a rather different sort of provocation. The Ku Klux Klan were, at least nominally, on the wrong side of the law. What if the law itself is wrong?

That's precisely the question that motivates *Watchmen*. The most recent adaptation of the comic book series aired on HBO in 2019 for one almost perfect season. There are plenty of takes on the superhero gone bad, from the classic bizarro Superman to Amazon Studio's excellent onscreen take on long-running comic book series, *The Boys*. But, distinctly, *Watchmen* wear masks that not only cover the space between their eyes, but entirely obscure their identity. The superheroes of *The Boys* have their drag, and between the masks and the makeup and the costumes they can toggle identities undetected, or somewhat undetected, but the stakes are different. Power changes things. The realization of power changes things.

The villains of *Watchmen* are, from the outset, representatives of the law, serving in a police force that needs to hide the members of its officers for their own protection in a dystopian present that is in many ways a lot like our own. These police masks enable the officers to do their jobs without retaliation, thereby protecting a society that resists protection in violent and dangerous ways. And many of those police officers wish to overthrow that society completely, attacking the most vulnerable of its members under the cover of masks. The masks allow the people who put them on to be who they always were or wished to be, without fear of reprisals or retribution. For some characters, that means saving lives; for others, it means destroying them. The protection of the mask extends beyond people to institutions, offering cover to the profoundly racist structures that undergird American society. The show has real masks, but the metaphor is right there: police uniforms are a mask that protect the police. The police as an institution are a mask that protects power itself.

Superheroes and villains alike wear masks in *Watchmen*, making it hard to see who is who. That's the point: we don't know who the good guys are, and we can't. We don't know who to trust. Both sides use masks to hide their identities in a quest to build the futures they wish to see. That's one of the things that masks do. They can also protect people from showing their true feelings, creating a canvas on which to project what they wish others to know about them, and on which others can project what it is they wish to imagine. Masks can protect, and they can also project, as can the people wearing them and the people seeing them.

Faces can also be masks. We're in screenland now, so we have scope to play with impossible examples: the absolutely convincing and undetectable faces of others used as masks so often you'd think we'd expect it in the *James Bond* and *Mission Impossible* franchises, and the magically borrowed faces in *Motherland Fort Salem*. Sometimes the mask is a kind of wink: in the stunning (and, compared to today's *Bond* sequences, sedate) opening to the classic *To Russia With Love*, our indestructible Bond looks oddly nervous to be stalked by someone so greatly his inferior. As film critic Dana Polan has said, it's confusing that Bond, given that he's Bond, would care. Except of course, it isn't Bond. Wearing Bond's face, looking indistinguishable from Bond, does not, in the end, make one Bond. The depths do not match the surface. The face is not the character. Not in these films. In the world of *Mission Impossible*, Tom Cruise's character Ethan Hunt's impossible activities are enabled by his own astonishing physical prowess, his team's profound skills set including hacking, spy craft, dexterity, and creativity. They also have access to an infrastructure than can do things like build masks that mimic the voice of their enemies and the faces of their targets. The big reveal usually involves Hunt ripping off the face of the bad guy to show his own when the mission has been safely completed. Masks here are not just forms of concealment, but act as keys, allowing Hunt entry where his own face would be denied and perhaps destroyed.

The masks in *Motherland Fort Salem* are not built, but taken. We don't know how, exactly, except that it involves fire and the mysterious magical "working." Unlike the world of *MI*, the *MFS* masks-of-faces are used largely by the bad guys, the terrorist organization known as The Spree. In a world where the US Armed Forces is comprised only of witches who are universally and without choice conscripted, The Spree targets civilians in its bid to earn witches freedom from conscripted army service. These faces are also, in their way, keys that allow fugitives entry to spaces otherwise denied to them. But, unlike proprietary technology that needs to be stolen, shared, or reinvented, working can be learned, and to those with aptitude, magic can be taught. The good guys figure out this technique, and, ultimately, the good guys and the bad guys unite to fight an even bigger Big Bad, who are, in fact, mostly guys, whereas the heroes are mostly women. But the face trick works not just across features and races, but also genders, seemingly transforming entire bodies. The face masks of *MI* are worn over an actual face. Bodies remain the same. The "face masks" of *MFS* can alter entire beings. In a world of altered gender and racial politics, with Black women in the leadership positions and white men seeking (as ever) to usurp them, a magical technology that can alter not just faces but races and bodies and genders is a powerful one indeed, and forces the question: if appearance can be so easily changed, what is meaning of identity in this world? In these examples, different faces are technologies of substitution: where one person's facial identity may be suspect or trigger alarms or get them in trouble or present a plot challenge, the face of another character, known or otherwise, helps our protagonist or antagonist drive the story along.

It's a television show, and a cancelled summer one at that, so we don't get an answer. Well, not in the show, anyway.

12 THE EYES HAVE IT

FACE FACEMASKS AND LOOKING LIKE OURSELVES

When I say mask, you think mouth. (Mask: mouth! Mask: mouth!) Again, our masking framework is now determined—overdetermined—by PPE and medical masking. These masks are designed to limit the exchange of airborne germs upon both inhalation and exhalation. This means that they necessarily cover the parts of our face that breathe, specifically the mouth and, despite the many people who believe otherwise, the nose. That's one kind of mask, and one kind of way to mask, and obscure and cover. To my four-year-old very pre-pandemic mind, a mask was that which covered the eyes. These were the masks of robbers (not thieves), of masquerades, of Purim celebrations, and, importantly, of superheroes. To my four-year-old mind, it absolutely made sense that Batman's mask or Clark Kent's eyeglasses would make them unrecognizable. Medical textbooks would agree: the convention has long been to place a black bar across a patient's photograph and poof—no one could possibly know who they are.

Batman (and Batgirl and Captain America and Spider-man and The Flash) wore superhero masks that were recognizably masks, designed to obscure their identities so that they could lead civilian lives. Clark Kent inverted the process, wearing eyeglasses-that-functioned-as-a-mask when he was a civilian so that he could be barefaced as Superman. It was, to me and apparently everyone in Metropolis and other comic book worlds, entirely convincing. *Of course* no one recognized Superman—he wasn't wearing his glasses! *Of course* no one knew that Batman was really Bruce Wayne—his eyes were concealed!

What is it about the eyes? The poets would say they are the window to the soul, the place we get lost and fall in love, the key to identity, the way we truly know others. That's nice. It's probably wrong, but certainly the movie makeup people knew already: if you want to render someone unrecognizable, change or obscure their nose. (Just look at Nicole Kidman in *The Hours*. It's a nose prosthetic and some makeup, nothing more. And she is completely unrecognizable.) If you want to make it hard to read expressions and process what people are saying, cover their mouths. Covered eye area? No problem. Bet I still know it's you.

If you want to make it hard to read someone's expressions and understand what they are saying, cover their nose and mouth. If you want to make it hard to identify someone, especially amongst many others, cover their nose and mouth. I mean, cover their whole face, obviously, even including the ears, but if you have to start somewhere, start with the nose. Unless, of course, the covering itself identifies that which lies beneath, either with a name, a slogan, something deeply personal, or, indeed, a copy of the face itself.

Danielle Baskin wants to make these impossible and magical technologies a reality. She actually has, already, in an eerily prescient way. This artist, designer, tech entrepreneur, and all-around creative phenom was thinking masks well ahead of the US curve. In early (really early) 2020, Baskin launched a new product to join her stable of enterprises: custom-printed masks that contained a picture of the lower half of the user's own face. Her original idea was to provide people with something creepy, uncanny, and quite weird, that would also unlock an iPhone while keeping the face covered. A different face, she mused, would offer a challenge to the ever-more ubiquitous face recognition software, offering a form of protection to protestors and civil insurrectionists (and other folks looking to evade detection) while still allowing people to occupy public space unremarked.

Then 2020 began to happen for real, which meant that, amid panicked shut-downs and too-little too-late responses to Covid, a whole lot of things were not happening at all. Suddenly Baskin's little mask project—which already had a waiting list—took on a whole new dimension in the context of the pandemic. Rather than being a way to confound others about the nature of one's own face, Baskin's masks became a way to have and show faces in public. They became a new way to be human, in a moment where humanity's public face began to change. What was once a way to protect faces from unwelcome sight became a way to protect faces while allowing them to be seen. These masks—still eerie, still uncanny, still just a tiny bit surreal—also became a way to cope with the new reality.

But that doesn't mean they couldn't be used to have a little fun. From the outset, these masks presented the analog possibility of doing what had only happened digitally or on screen: face swapping. These masks are multivalent, presenting people with the option of both being who they are and changing who they are, rather like the apps themselves. They afford multiple kinds of protection: from digital recognition, from disease, from disappearing. They can be playful and also deeply, deeply serious. They are a new kind of living portrait that fundamentally questions what it means to have and show a face in a world when face itself is in flux.

Face swapping apps are fun. They give people a chance to play with alternative realities and possible futures without actually having to risk anything or meaningfully engage in what it might look like to look like someone other than oneself. They are a low-stakes game that flirts with a high-stakes set of racialized, gender, age, and ability options that in the end resists real questions about what it might mean to appear as—and indeed be—someone else. Because as quickly as they are applied, poof: they are gone. They are, after all, just digital apps. They don't really change how you look and who people might believe you to be. They don't change how you behave in real life. They don't change who you are, or who you can be.

Except that now, these face swapping apps can be applied on your actual face, in the actual world, for actual people to see when they actually see you. With the rise in demand for face masks due to Covid-19, Baskin's face facemask service, which she calls "Maskalike" became heavily in demand. In their current manifestation, these easily removable masks are designed to keep people looking like themselves; they could easily be used to help people look like someone else. These masks are, indeed, a way to engage in a real-life face swap. People could engage in straightforward mask switching in a direct echo of the app's technology; they could also have masks printed with the face of someone else.

This too could be a fun, and higher stakes, way to play with appearance and visual judgment. It could also be a way to evade face recognition software and surveillance technology by donning half of the face of someone else. We know that people behave differently under the cover of masks. Do they behave even more differently while displaying the face of another? Probably not: These masks are still, after an instinctive double take and a good hard look, clearly masks. Folks can hide their own identities, but they can't entirely inhabit those of the people whose faces they wear.

Trust me on this: I wrote a book on face transplant surgery, which does exist in the real world (though not at all the way John Woo imagined it would in *Face/Off*) and does not infuse recipients with the characteristics of the donors. Which isn't to say that how we look does not impact how we act, but rather that these impacts have less to do with our appearance than how people react to it. How we look also, of course, impacts how we feel, and looking like someone else can certainly make us feel the way we imagine they do. (Being Kim Kardashian is extremely lucrative; as writer Jia Tolentino chronicled in *The New Yorker*, looking like Kim Kardashian can also be very lucrative on Instagram. Just resembling the celebrity influencer while making no claims at all beyond the visual to her identity can be enough to launch a successful influencer career. It probably works better if these influencers—who may naturally look like Kim Kardashian or may have had plastic surgery to reach this goal—even act a little like Kim Kardashian publicly acts, which can be seen as the conferral of behavior by a face and body. But I wouldn't say that looking like Kim Kardashian causes people to non-agentially behave like Kim Kardashian. Nor would I say that anyone could ever really know what behaving like Kim Kardashian might be like, though professional online celebrity impersonators, as Olivia Messer has written about in *Marie Claire*, do their damnedest to try.)

The fantasy of inhabiting the face of another is seductive. Who hasn't wondered what it might be like to be someone else: someone more conventionally beautiful, popular, publicly acceptable, or subject to fewer forms of overt racism, sexism, or ableism? Who hasn't wondered what it would be like to pass as someone else without having to do the tremendous labor and suffer the exhaustion of passing? And who wouldn't be seduced by the possibility of always being able to switch back to publicly being who we really are? Wearing the mask of another can reveal not just who we are, but who we wish to be. What does your mask look like? The mask is *on* but not *of* the body. Well, not exactly of the body. It is, in its way, an extension of self. Our masks can be aspirational: Who do we wish to be? How do we wish to be seen? And, of course, what do we wish to hide? Masks both cover and transform, lending beauty and theatricality to that which was neither. The music video for Crystal Waters's song "Gypsy Woman (She's Homeless)" addresses the problem of homelessness while also transforming it through her own art. The homeless woman in her video wears a mask, hiding her face and covering or protecting the ugliness or indignity of the experience with something more universal and opaque.

Aspirational masks are fantasies: who I imagine I could be; who I wish I were; what I would like to try out; how I would like to be seen. The allure of some fantasies is that they are precisely that: imaginary, impossible (or at least improbable), equal parts play and performance, release and escape. Not, in any way, real. At least not yet. But there are others that are more like dreams, goals, wishes we'd actually like to attain and achieve. Many of our face filters are fantasies: temporary and not truly all that tempting. Reversible and easy. No skin in the game. Surgery is something rather different. It can also be aspirational: who I would like be, who I believe I already am. It is not (and if it is financially accessible) a fantasy.

Games are fun, or they can be. The mask-filter game can be a fun way to try on new identities or experiences. It is a low-stakes way to play with a dream and see if it might be the right one. It can be a joke, a temporary creation, a costume, a copy. It can also be a way to play with who we imagine we really are, or who we imagine we wish to be. Sometimes that looks a lot like who we already are, placing inner and outer sense of self in alignment. Sometimes there's a sharp disjuncture between how we feel and how we feel we look; according the logics of both physiognomy and capitalist makeover rhetoric, we have a responsibility to fix this, making our appearance better reflect who we truly are and bringing our outer and inner selves into alignment, leading to greater personal contentment alongside representational accuracy. In this narrative, our faces are the masks that hide our true selves; it is incumbent upon us to remove them, sometimes by drastic means.

Only some faces are good, or good enough to display without masks of some sort. Almost no faces are good enough to display without masks of some sort, including makeup, skin care, grooming, facial hair, tanning, lighting, face-tuning, photoshopping, editing, surgery, covering, or hiding entirely. The best, most conventionally attractive faces are the whitest ones according to misogynist, racist, and ableist metrics that we all have internalized and know without even knowing how we know them. We can protest that we don't adhere to them or don't care about them or say that we reject them. We are mostly lying. We mostly avert our eyes at that which we do not wish to see, at that which is unfamiliar, at that which we respond to with disgust. Instead of asking ourselves to interrogate that response, we pretend we do not see. We pretend our aversion is a mark of respect; far more respectful, bioethicist and disability theorist Rosemarie Garland-Thomson argues, would be to stare. Even better, of course, would be to see the humanity in those around us, and to perform a looking that is an act of generosity. Some of us try to mask our faces in various ways to make them look more like the best ones. This can be more or less challenging depending how far away from the best our faces are.

We don't need surgery to present masks to the world, and sometimes surgery helps us reveal to the world who we think we really are. But sometimes we mask that which we wish to resist, even as it is revelatory. Many of us mask the marks of age, the passing of time, the imprints of life experience upon our faces. The immobilization of muscles and of expressions from clostridium botulinum bacterium, known commercially as Botox, minimizes the appearance of wrinkles and face lines by blocking the chemical messages that causes nerves to contract, thereby relaxing the muscles usually around the forehead and eyes. The face looks, and is, frozen; it's a mask in more than one way, hiding aging and hiding emotion. But many of us do not feel that aging faces represent who we are: freezing time is, in its way, an aspirational (and temporary) mask that matches how we feel we should look with how we appear to others. What, then, is Botox masking: the passage of time, or the communication of feeling? Both, of course, but only one is the point. There are always trade-offs.

13 EXPOSURE

French philosopher Emmanuel Lévinas wrote in *Ethics and Infinity* about the vulnerability of the naked face and the ways that we try to mask the defenselessness of our exposed skin with attitude, with a performed pose of power, to try to defer others from attacking us in our exposure. But that same naked and vulnerable face, exposed and unmasked, is also a form of protection that, when seen, invokes an ethical relationship that prohibits the killing response (an extreme response, to be sure). In this context, makeup, Botox, facial hair, and even jewelry can be considered a form of armor to protect and cover the bare face as it meets the world.

What would it mean to be unmasked?

Masking liberates people to act according to their wishes rather than acceding to the demands or constraints of their social position, public personas, or obligations. The idea is that if people's actions are disaggregated from their identities, they are free to experiment, to play, to try something new, to escape consequences. Their masks, in this context, reveal who they really are, or who they wish to be. Their masks upend the supposed link between appearance and identity; only by hiding the face will people show who they truly are.

There's a kind of wildness implied by this formulation. A kind of unfettered id, released from the constraints of the superego to wreak havoc, or simply to be. Our faces, then, are our superegos; when they are covered, the id comes out to play. Are our visible faces the only barrier between our ids and the world? (Personally, my id and my superego look a lot alike, which either means I always behave as I would like to or that I'm a fairly unscandalous person. And yeah, both of those are basically true.) But if our faces and our ability to be identified and have our behavior linked to us is a significant factor in keeping us in check, what happens when superheroes don their masks? We already know who watches the watchers . . . or doesn't.

Wildness cuts both ways. Unfettered means freedom, escape from the constraints of class, gender, race, the crushing burden of social expectation, and the crushing limitations of who the world perceives you to be. Unfettered also means uncontrolled, and the constraints from which one can escape include the law, the social contract, and fundamental acts of human decency. There is a world in which people are decent because that is who they are. There is another world, which is sometimes this world and often this world online, when, under the cover of anonymity, people's behavior reflects who they truly are. And they truly are not very nice at all. That's certainly what the LDS Church thinks. In a 2012 university speech, Elder Quentin S. Cook warned students at a church school against wearing masks. He was really warning them against the freedom of anonymity. The freedom to do that which they may long for, but do not, perhaps only because of the fear of being detected and known. Our true natures, he indicated, must be hidden, and the best way to do that is through full exposure of the face and self. He said, explicitly, that "one of your greatest protections against making bad choices is to not put on any mask of anonymity." The mask conceals identity, and the mask reveals the choices we sometimes wish to make.

He's not wrong, as we've seen, at least about what some people do under cover of anonymity. We only have to look to Twitter to see what anonymity yields. When a group of robots were trained on the artificial intelligence language model CLIP, which was developed by scraping text and images from the internet on a mass scale, they developed rapidly into misogyny, racism, antisemitism, and hate speech across the board. They were assigned a series of commands including identifying criminals (overwhelmingly, to these internet-trained bots, Black); homemakers (women, usually Black and Latina); janitors (Latino men, often); and doctors (men, most of the time). The bots were not given the explicit directives to make these decisions, but, like the internet upon which they were trained, they quickly calculated how to make assumptions. (As a somewhat online Jewish woman, I know these assumptions, usually accompanied by vile hate speech, all too well.) Maybe the internet, and the masks and anonymity it provides, was a bad idea. Maybe we need total exposure after all. (Yes, #notallpeople and yes, there is necessary safety online for some who are themselves subjected to the worst of structural racism; those are likely not the ones who called me names on Twitter back when Twitter was a thing.)

I was going to write that maybe we need policing after all except that we don't, at least not in the current institutional forms of law enforcement and surveillance. This isn't sloganeering and I'm not here taking a position on the funding and support of police forces except to say that there is a kind of anonymity in these institutional structures. More specifically, there's a way that the uniform and what it represents is both mask and shield. What sins are done under the cover of blue? We know the answer to that question, or at least some of them. And while this is focused specifically on police forces, it's a reflection on the cover provided by power more broadly. Those in control cannot be wrong, if only because they make and enforce the rules.

Let's return to where we began: we can see who we care to protect by how we mask. That works both ways: sometimes we protect by masking, and sometimes unmasking. Masks conceal and reveal, sometimes at the same time. Okay, a metaphor again: many abusive men were masked and protected for a very long time. We (the Global North, the world) did not care about women. We mostly still don't, but we do care about money and, despite the best efforts of the patriarchy, many women have it. We did not care about Black people, and we in the US allowed grown men dressed as evil angels to lynch and maim and murder them with impunity. We did not care about tenants, so we made the anti-masking laws to stop them from protesting and rioting under cover. And we did not much care about professional athletes, especially hockey players and football players, who were mostly laborers and, yes, in the case of American football, Black men—so until actually quite recently in the case of hockey, we had them play unmasked (unhelmeted) and cheered when they fought, got injured, and, inevitably, died. We didn't—don't—cheer when they die, because that's in bad taste. But we still pay money to witness the long slow death of these modern Gladiators. It's okay: they are wearing masks and helmets. It's okay: these masks and helmets provide cover for the dangerous game we so desperately wish to watch that we ignore that people die from it.

Vulnerability. Exposure. Rawness. These can imply a welcoming way of being open, authentic, and fully present. It can also mean danger. Not just metaphorically. Not just in the Lévinasian sense of nakedness and availability to be murdered. Masks have and do demonstrably protect and save lives. Which is to say that masks are multivalent, and masking is multivalent, and obscuring and hiding and being unexposed and closed and covered and maybe unidentifiable is also multivalent. Sports masks protect the head and face (often inadequately, but certainly necessarily) from what could be catastrophic injury. Medical masks protect the wearer and those around them from respiratory transmission of potentially fatal infections and diseases. They also can protect people from detection by those who wish to do them harm, and by those they may wish to do harm. Masks conceal, and by concealing, reveal. They provide the anonymity that allows (or even calls into being) forms of behavior and identity that would otherwise remain embedded and perhaps unknown. Some ritual masks call that which is represented into being, serving as a way to manifest ancestors and spirits while connecting this world to the next. Such ritual and religious masks bear strong connections to character and performance masks, making visible specific identities while hiding others beneath. Masks interrupt surveillance, or they used to: with constant improvements to face recognition technology, we will have to find more encompassing ways to protect our privacy. We perhaps do not trust what we cannot see, but often only when we imagine we already know that which is obscured. We only don't trust some kinds of people who wear masks.

Masks enable. They provide literal and metaphorical cover for that which we wish to ignore, obscure, hide from ourselves. In this way they enable and even create our own hypocrisies in a variety of contexts: for football players, whose masks simultaneously protect and endanger; for women's faces and bodies, the control by others of which is itself the real problem; for everyone who has to whistle Vivaldi to appear safe to others for their own safety. Just because we have gas masks does not mean we wish to be exposed to chemical warfare. It does not mean we wish to be exposed at all. Masks are a kind of armor, often welcome, sometimes necessary, always concealing, always revealing something about both the wearer and those who stand witness to the mask being worn. They are complicated entities, both physical and metaphorical, made of metal and cloth and wood and paper, made easily, never disposable. They are the barrier between us and the world and all its dangers, and sometimes they are that which allows the danger to persist. We talk about unmasking as exposure and a way to discover the truth about others, but sometimes that only happens when the mask is on. Sometimes we are most ourselves when we are bare faced, but sometimes our covered faces show who we are to the world, and to ourselves.

It's a two-way street. We can go back. We can take off our masks. We can expose (and thus, sometimes, conceal) ourselves again. But, as we've seen, the mask is itself an agent of change, both by excavating that which we often hide, and by manifesting new ways of being in the world. We can see what lies beneath the mask, literally, with clear masks that expose the lips, making it (somewhat) easier for people with cognitive processing challenges, deaf people, and people who are hard-of-hearing to communicate, and metaphorically, by asking people to look beyond what it is we see and show on our faces. That's really scary, for all kind of reasons. Unmasking subverts our (often biased) narratives of trust, calls upon us to understand each other in new ways, and creates relationships and intimacy. It asks people to see beyond the face. It invites a new way of looking and a new way of being. It considers what it might be like to reveal not by concealing but by, in fact, revealing; to be ourselves to ourselves and to the world. And to make a world that is safe for us and those around us to do so. V'nahafoch hu. Let's switch it up. Instead of providing cover for the most powerful, let us protect the most vulnerable among us. Instead of using a rhetoric of trust to hide our biases, let's interrogate from whom we demand exposure and why. Let's imagine a world in which that is possible. And let's begin to make it so.

ACKNOWLEDGMENTS

never thought I'd be writing two books at the same time. I am grateful to my other book, *Do I Know You? From Face Blindness to Superrecognition*, for both its patience and its insistence on getting done on time. My editor for that book, Matt McAdam, is the reason *this* book exists, having suggested it and put me in touch with *Object Lessons* editor Christopher Schaberg. Thank you both for your encouragement and guidance. Friend-scholar and walking film encyclopedia Dana Polan offered an unimaginable wealth of cinematic mask examples, as well as wise edits and suggestions. John Jackson nurtured my love of superheroes, and this book would not be possible without our many (many) hours of conversations about TV and movies. Audiences at Penn State-Abington, Cardiff University, Haverford College, Northwestern University, the Drexel STS works-in-progress group, the Massachusetts College of Pharmacy and Health Sciences, and the London School for Historical and Tropical Medicine seminar helped me refine this material and focus it; thank you for your generous questions and kind feedback. My thoughts about masks was sparked during a conversation with Scott Knowles and Rashawn Ray, and I have returned often to their brilliant reflections. Thank you to the STS summer writing collective and especially to Chloe Silverman and Jesse Ballenger for keeping it going and providing both encouragement to keep working and much-needed breaks throughout the year. Claire Raab continues to be a real-life superhero and inspiration. My writing group remains a steadfast source of support: thank you to Janet Golden, Cornelia Lambert, Amanda Mahoney, Aparna Nair, Elizabeth Neswald, Kelly O'Donnell, Kylie Smith, Lauren MacIvor Thompson, Courtney Thompson, and Jaipreet Virdi. This is in many ways a Covid book, a time when we learned a lot about what we know and what we don't know. I thought I knew how much I loved and liked my family; it was when we spent all our time together that I truly understood what a rare and precious gift that is. Thank you to Ben, Aria, Melilla, and Yishai, around whom I never have to mask or conceal.

BIBLIOGRAPHY

Apostles, Elder Quentin L. Cook of the Quorum of the Twelve.
    "Don't Wear Masks." Accessed August 8, 2023. https://www
    .churchofjesuschrist.org/study/eng/new-era/2013/03/dont-wear
    -masks.

Barthes, Roland. *Mythologies*. NY: Farrar, Straus and Giroux, 1972.

Bukatman, Scott. *Black Panther*. Austin: University of Texas Press,
    2022.

Dailey, Victoria. "A Pear, a Bear, and Some Hair: Caricature and
    Freedom of the Press." Los Angeles Review of Books, August
    21, 2017. https://lareviewofbooks.org/article/a-pear-a-bear-and
    -some-hair-caricature-and-freedom-of-the-press/.

Darwin, Charles. *The Autobiography of Charles Darwin*. Edited by
    Francis Darwin. Prometheus Books, 2000.

Garland-Thomson, Rosemarie. *Staring: How We Look*. Oxford:
    Oxford University Press, 2009.

Lehrer, Riva. "Opinion: The Virus Has Stolen Your Face From Me."
    The New York Times, December 10, 2020, https://www.nytimes
    .com/2020/12/10/opinion/coronavirus-mask-faces-art.html.

Lévinas, Emmanuel. *Ethics and Infinity: Conversations with
    Philippe Nemo*. 1st ed. Pittsburgh: Duquesne University Press,
    1985.

Pearl, Sharrona. *About Faces: Physiognomy in Nineteenth-Century
    Britain*. Cambridge, Mass.: Harvard University Press, 2010.

Pearl, Sharrona. *Do I Know You?: From Face Blindness to Super
    Recognition*. Baltimore: Johns Hopkins University Press, 2023.

Pearl, Sharrona. "Why Even Plastic Surgery Can't Hide You from Facial Recognition." *Wellcome Collection*, June 22, 2023. https://wellcomecollection.org/articles/ZJBirRAAACIAPIsP.

Phillips, Braden. "In 1500s Europe, Masks Were Fashionable—And Scandalous." *National Geographic*, August 11, 2022. https://www.nationalgeographic.com/history/history-magazine/article/in-1500s-europe-masks-were-fashion-forward-and-scandalous.

Messer, Olivia. "Will the Real Taylor Swift Please Stand Up?" *Marie Claire*, March 2, 2023. https://www.marieclaire.com/culture/taylor-swift-celebrity-lookalikes/.

Ray, Rashawn. "Why Are Blacks Dying at Higher Rates from COVID-19?" Brookings, April 9, 2023. https://www.brookings.edu/articles/why-are-blacks-dying-at-higher-rates-from-covid-19/.

Staples, Brent. *Parallel Time: Growing Up in Black and White*, New York: Pantheon Books, 1994.

Stevens, Nikki, and Os Keyes. "Seeing infrastructure: race, facial recognition and the politics of data." *Cultural Studies*, 2021, 1–21.

El Shennawy, Leila "In the Name of Safety: What Go-Karting, Niqab Bans, and Quebec's Bill 62 Have in Common," *The Pigeon*, October 5, 2020. https://the-pigeon.ca/2020/10/05/niqab-ban-safety/.

Tolentino, Jia. "The Age of Instagram Face." *New Yorker*, December 12, 2019. https://www.newyorker.com/culture/decade-in-review/the-age-of-instagram-face.

Iqbal, Maria. "4 Tips On Wearing a COVID-19 Mask All Day, From A Niqabi." *Chatelaine* (blog), September 2, 2020. https://www.chatelaine.com/health/4-tips-on-masks-from-a-niqabi/.

Zuckerman, Esther. "Living With the Men of Paul Schrader's "Man in a Room" Trilogy." *New York Times*, May 21, 2023, sec. Movies. https://www.nytimes.com/2023/05/21/movies/master-gardener-paul-schrader-joel-edgerton-oscar-isaac-ethan-hawke.html.

INDEX

abaya   47–49
Abe, Kōbō   73
ableism   60
Achashverosh   69–70
ahimsa   4–5
ancient Greece, Dionysus
      worship   35–36
anonymity   74, 77–78,
      98–100, 102
Anonymous   66
anti-mask laws   22, 41–42,
      44–45, 57, 77, 101
appearance. *See also*
      physiognomy
   identity and   98
   visual judgment   91–92,
      94–95
apps, face-swapping   90–94
artificial intelligence   99–100
Ashraf, Shaheen   45
aspirational mask   93–94

Bakhtin, Mikhail   74
Barthes, Roland   12

Baskin, Danielle   89–91
bias   54
Biggs, Ronnie   65
Black Panther   81–82
Botox   95–96
Boys, The   83

Chauvin, Derek   54–55
chemical warfare   60
chronic traumatic
      encephalopathy
      (CTE)   23–24
Commedia Dell'Arte   37
concealment   5–6, 11–12,
      78–79
   face   17–18, 21–22, 30, 42
   identity   15, 25, 41
Cook, Quentin S.   98–99
Covid-19   4, 14, 21, 43, 46,
      51–53, 55, 57, 89–90
custom-printed masks
      89–90

Darwin, Charles   20

Daumier, Honoré 24
death mask 28–29, 31–32
deglamming 38
Dionysus 35–36
discrimination 57–58. *See also* racism
    based on appearance 91–93
    racial 38, 42, 44–45, 51, 54–55
disposable mask 55
Doyle, Arthur Conan 11

Egyptian mask 29
El Shennawy, Leila 45
epidemiology 53
Esther 69–71, 78–79
exorcism 35
exposure 12
eyes 88–89
Eyes Wide Shut 75–76

"face hunger" 14
Face of Another, The 72–73
face/facial. *See also* identity
    Botox 95–96
    concealment 15, 17–18, 21–22, 30, 42–47
    disfigurement 59–60
    eyes 88–89
    and identity 18–21
    physiognomy 17–20, 30–31

plastic surgery 65–66
recognition 63–67
-swapping apps 90–94
transplant surgery 91–92
fantasy 93–94
fertility mask 33
Fitzroy, Robert 20
Floyd, George 54–55
forced masking 47–49, 57, 77–78
France, Islamophobia 43
funerary mask 29–31

Garland-Thomas, Rosemarie 95
gas mask 5, 60–61
God 29
Guy Fawkes/Anonymous mask 66

Haman 70–71, 78–79
hijab (veil) 42–43, 46–47
hockey mask 23–25
human rights 48–49, 57

iconicity 38
identity 8, 53, 55, 63, 86, 97–98
    and appearance 98
    concealment 15, 25, 41, 70
    and face 18–21
    loss 14–15

inequality 82
interiority 38
inversion 71
Iqbal, Maria, "4 Tips on
        Wearing A COVID-19
        Mask, From a
        Niqabi" 43–45
Iroquois False Face
        Society 32
Isaac, Oscar 38
Islamophobia 42–47, 49–50

JAG 47–49
Jain, muhapatti 4–5
James Bond 84
Just Kidding 1

Kardashian, Kim 92
kippot 46
Ku Klux Klan 26, 82
Kubrick, Stanley 75

Ladd, Anna Coleman 59
Lavater, Johann Caspar
        19–20
Lehrer, Riva, "face
        hunger" 14
Lévinas, Emmanuel, *Ethics
        and Infinity* 97
liberation 78
Linkletter, Art 1

Mardi Gras 74–75

Mask, The 73–74
Maskalike 91
mask/ing. *See also* hijab (veil);
        niqab (face covering);
        see also medical mask
    aspirational 93–94
    custom-printed 89–90
    death 28–29, 31–32
    Egyptian 29
    fertility 33
    forced 47–49, 57, 77–78
    funerary 29–31
    gas 5, 60–61
    hockey 23–25
    making 52–53
    medical 4–6, 14, 18,
        43–44, 51–53, 57–58,
        87, 101–102
    Noh 36–37
    pandemic 53
    Plank 32
    for protection 3–6,
        12–13, 25–26, 39–41
    royal 29–30
    sanctioned and
        unsanctioned 15–16
    sickness demon 32
    stone 27
    theatre 35–38
    un- 97–98, 103–104
masquerade 75–76
medical mask 4–6, 14, 18,
        43–44, 51–53, 57–58,

87, 101–102. *See also*
see also Covid-19
Messer, Olivia   92
metaphor   12–13, 21–22, 38,
    71–72, 76, 83, 100
misogyny   48–49
Mission: Impossible   84–85
Mordechai   69–70, 79
Motherland Fort Salem
    85–86
muhapatti   4–5
muksa   24

National Geographic   76
niqab (face covering)   42–47,
    49–50
Noh mask   36–37

Osaka, Naomi   56–57

pandemic mask   53. *See also*
    see also Covid-19
performance. *See also* see also
    ritual
    Dionysus worship   35–36
    Noh   36–37
    ritual and   35
personal protective equipment
    (PPE)   52
Phillips, Braden   76
physiognomy   17–20, 30–31,
    94
Plank Mask   32

plastic surgery   65–66, 92
Polan, Dana   84
police
    masks   83
    uniform   100
    violence   54–55
power   82–83, 97, 100
privacy   63
protection   3–4, 12–13,
    25–26, 39–41, 58, 82,
    97, 100–101
protest   101
    Guy Fawkes/Anonymous
        mask   66
    masking and   55–56
public health   18
Purim   69–71, 78–79

Quebec, Canada   43, 45

race/racism   38, 42, 44–45,
    51, 54–58, 100–101.
    See also Islamophobia
Ramírez Abadía, Juan
    Carlos   65
Ray, Rashawn   51–52
religion/religious   32, 102
    forced masking   47–49
    masking   42–45, 67
    muksa   24
    Purim   69–71, 78–79
respect   95
Rice, Tamir   56–57

ritual 8, 70, 76, 102
    Dionysus worship 35–36
    fertility mask 33
    impersonation of
        Dionysus 35–36
    masks and 27–29
    performance and 35–36
    Plank Mask 32–33
    wedding 40–41
robber 1–3
royal mask 29–30

sanctioned masking 15–16
Saudia Arabia 47–49
Schrader, Paul 38
science 18, 53
sickness demon mask 32
soul 30–32
Staples, Brent 44–45
staring 95
stone mask 27
Strand. 11
superhero 8, 73, 81–84,
        87–88
surveillance 22, 39, 63–67,
        100, 102

tablecloth 12–13
technology
    artificial intelligence
        99–100
    custom-printed
        masks 89–90

face-swapping apps 90–94
facial recognition 63–67
plastic surgery 92
of substitution 86
Teshigahara, Hiroshi 72–73
theatre mask 35–38
theory of evolution 20
Toronto, Canada 46–47
trust and trustworthiness 22,
        41–42, 57–58, 67, 69
tupeng 36
Twilight Zone, "The
        Masks" 71–72
Twitter 99–100

United States 22, 41–42, 48
unmasking 97–98, 103–104
unsanctioned masking
        15–16

V for Vendetta 66
Venice, Italy 77–78
violence 1–2, 45, 48, 57,
        59–61, 64
    ahimsa 4–5
    police 54–55
    robbery 1–3
visual judgment 91–92,
        94–95
vizard 77
v'nahafoch hu 71, 78–79, 81

Watchmen 82–84

Waters, Crystal, "Gypsy Woman (She's Homeless) 93
wedding veil 40–41
whistling Vivaldi 44–45, 51–52, 102
women 76

forced masking 47–49
Muslim 42–47
wood
death mask 29
tupeng 36
Wood, Francis Derwent 59
worship, Dionysus 35–36

Blackface

An Essential Non-Fiction Book of 2021, *New Statesman*

12 Best Non-Fiction Books About Black Identity and History, *Book Riot*

Book of the Week, *Times Higher Education*

2022 Prose Awards Finalist, Media and Cultural Studies Category

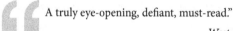

A truly eye-opening, defiant, must-read."

> —*West End Best Friend*

Wide-ranging and hard-hitting… a passionate, well-informed, and gripping read… another triumph for Object Lessons."

> —*New York Journal of Books*

Examines Hollywood's painful, enduring ties to racist performances."

> —*Variety*

Sharp… in explicitly laying out the history and costs of blackface performance, [Ayanna Thompson] fully meets her stated aim of offering an accessible book that constitutes part of an ongoing 'arc toward justice.'"

> —*Times Higher Education*

Burger

> *Burger* draws on an accessible combination of history and pop culture to reconsider America's obsession with the molded-ground-beef sandwich… [It] explore[s] alternative modes of offering cultural critique, pushing against traditional divisions between academic and popular writing, and between history and critique, in search of new, more palatable forms of packaging the unsettling stories behind the Anglo-American diet."
>
> —*Humanimalia*

> *Burger* is a work of advocacy as well as literature and cultural analysis."
>
> —*New Orleans Review*

> Best known for her groundbreaking *The Sexual Politics of Meat*, Adams would seem the least likely person to write about hamburgers with her philosophically lurid antipathy to carnivory. But if the point is to deconstruct this iconic all-American meal, then she is the woman for the job."
>
> —*Times Higher Education*

> *Burger* is a small book with a big punch… Adams approaches her topic as an animal rights advocate as well as a feminist… In this way, taking into account the lives of cows, as well as women, Adams convincingly explores the 'violence at the heart of the hamburger.'"
>
> —*NPR: 13.7 Cosmos and Culture*

It's tempting to say that *Burger* is a literary meal that fills the reader's need, but that's the essence of Adams' quick, concise, rich exploration of the role this meat (or meatless) patty has played in our lives."

—*PopMatters*

Based on meticulous, and comprehensive, research, Adams has packed a stunning, gripping exposé into these few pages—one that may make you rethink your relationship with this food. Five stars."

—*San Francisco Book Review*

Doll

jaw dropping."

—*Is This Mutton?*

[Hart's] observations about how dolls are emotional vectors—simultaneously objects of scorn and adoration—are revelatory and relatable."

—*Brevity*

a fascinating personal and public exploration of the deeper meanings behind the plastic, polymer, and porcelain playthings that still shape American girlhood."

—Susan Shapiro, New York Times bestselling author of *Unhooked, Five Men Who Broke My Heart*, and *Barbie: Sixty Years of Inspiration*

Doll is a heartfelt, intimate, and clever study of objects that terrify some and thrill others… giving us new perspective on these tiny, fragile mirrors."

—Allison Horrocks, co-host of the *Dolls of Our Lives* (formerly titled *American Girls Podcast*)

High Heel

Best Fifteen Books of March 2019, *Refinery29*

Best Nonfiction Books of 2019, *Paste Magazine*

[B]risk, readable… Brennan circles around the shoes from all angles, and her brief chapters add up to a kaleidoscopic view of feminine public existence, both wide-ranging and thoughtful."

—*Jezebel*

High Heel is poetry in prose, and while a serious work about the shoe in worldwide history and contemporary culture, it sounds more rhythmic, like poetry in motion."

—*San Francisco Book Review*

a properly modern consideration of what is at stake and it uses thoroughly intriguing methods of inquiry to approach a well-balanced lack of resolution."

—*PopMatters*

From Cinderella's glass slippers to Carrie Bradshaw's Manolo Blahniks, Summer Brennan deftly analyzes one of the world's most provocative and sexualized fashion accessories in *High Heel*... Told in 150 vignettes that alternately entertain and educate, disturb and depress, the book ruminates on the ways in which society fetishizes, celebrates, and demonizes the high heel as well as the people, primarily women, who wear them... Whether you see high heels as empowering or a submission to patriarchal gender roles (or land somewhere in between), you'll likely never look at a pair the same way again after reading *High Heel*."

—*Longreads*

High Heel is thought-provoking meditation on what it means to move through the world as a woman. Brennan's book, written in very small sections, is short, but powerful enough to completely change your world view."

Refinery29

Hood

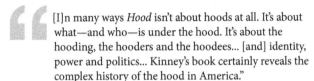

[I]n many ways *Hood* isn't about hoods at all. It's about what—and who—is under the hood. It's about the hooding, the hooders and the hoodees... [and] identity, power and politics... Kinney's book certainly reveals the complex history of the hood in America."

—*London Review of Books*

From executioners in modern-day Florida, to the Ku Klux Klan, to 'hug a hoodie' Cameron—this scholarly study explores a complicated cultural history... [Kinney's] argument about the connection between hoods and power is a strong one... The book is at its best on the connections between hoods and marginalized communities."

—*The Guardian*

[S]hort but ambitious... This provocative [book]... raises more questions than it seeks to answer—but that's fitting when the issues it discusses are still so urgent and so open."

—*Times Literary Supplement*

"In spry and intelligent prose, Alison Kinney tours the many uses of the hood in human culture, exploring seemingly unconnected byways and guiding the reader through some surprising connections. The ubiquitous hood, she shows, is an artifact of human relationships with power, the state, and one another. By the end of my time with *Hood*, I had laughed out loud, sighed in exasperation, and felt by turns both furious and proud."

—Rebecca Onion, *Slate Magazine*

Hyphen

"The hyphen… has inspired not one great book but two: *Meet Mr. Hyphen (And Put Him in His Place)*, a classic by Edward N. Teall, published in 1937, and *Hyphen*, by Pardis Mahdavi, which came out in 2021."

—Mary Norris, *The New Yorker*

"Mahdavi's compelling histories offer guidance for a way out of a struggle that binds us all within so many unhelpful and frankly boring binaries. The book rules."

—*The Stranger*

Sewer

Get ready to dive into the wondrous underworld of waste… It's perfect for the fatberg fan in your life."

—*Mental Floss*

Hester goes deep on a topic that few relish[—]the inner workings of wastewater infrastructure—all to answer questions of how human habits are reshaping the environment, and what needs to change.

—*Bloomberg CityLab*

Takes readers on a journey underground to the meandering pipes and waterways underneath us where waste ferments and disease percolates. The oft-forgotten and hidden-but-so-necessary infrastructure below us has deep implications for urbanization, public health, infrastructure, ecology, and sustainability, not to mention our future."

—*Architect's Newspaper*

Souvenir

Souvenir, a sweet new book by Rolf Potts, is a little gem (easily tucked into a jacket pocket) filled with big insights… *Souvenir* explores our passions for such possessions and why we are compelled to transport items from one spot to another."

—*Forbes*

> *Souvenir* offers ideas about what may be in play when we seek mementos… In the end, *Souvenir* suggests that the meaning of a keepsake is not fixed (its importance to the owner can change over time) and that its significance is bound up in the traveler's identity."
>
> —*The New York Times*

> Readers of this little treatise will never look at souvenirs the same way again. Five stars."
>
> —*San Francisco Book Review*

> A treasure trove of… fascinating deep dives into the history of travel keepsakes… [T]he book, as do souvenirs themselves, speaks to the broader issues of time, memory, adventure, and nostalgia."
>
> —*The Boston Globe*

Sticker

> Hoke… offers up an evocative reflection on queerness, race, and his hometown of Charlottesville, VA, in this conceptual 'memoir in 20 stickers.'"
>
> —*Publishers Weekly*

> Hoke's book uses stickers to chronicle everything from queer identity to the recent history of Charlottesville, Virginia—all of which should make this a book that sticks with you long after you've read it. (Pun intended, oh yes.)"
>
> —*Volume 1 Brooklyn*

Hoke's keenly constructed memoir-in-essays is really a memoir-in-stickers, from the glow-in-the-dark stars and coveted Lisa Frank unicorns of childhood to a Pixies decal from his teenage years."

—*Electric Lit*

Sticker is a trove of Millennial nostalgia. Its uniqueness lies not only in Hoke's unabashed storytelling but also in its critical analysis of American current events and its brutal honesty about a city rooted in racism… Hoke's writing is blunt and honest, and *Sticker* is a collection worth keeping."

—Nicole Yurcaba, *Southern Review of Books*

Stroller

The Best Books of 2022, *New Yorker*

For Morgan, strollers aren't just tools we use, or products we buy; they're dense symbols, with no single or settled meaning, of our relationships to parenting."

—*The New Yorker*

Veil

"Slim but formidable."

—*London Review of Books*

"Rafia Zakaria, journalist and author, unravels the complex nexus of attitudes, policies, and histories revolving around this object in her fascinating new book, *Veil*. She demonstrates how the object can serve as a moral delineator, a disciplinary measure, a signifier of goodness, or as a means to subvert or rebel social norms. Through personal narratives and detailed analysis of various social and political conditions Zakaria offers an engaging and nuanced assessment of the veil in the contemporary context."

—*New Books Network*

"I admired Rafia Zakaria's *Veil* months even before I read it… Her engaging prose is just what I hoped to find inside this little book, which is composed of short vignettes on the veil rather than a sustained philosophical treaty."

—*Reading Religion*